Praise For Book

"This book should be required reading for every lupus patient. After following this program for six months, I am no longer taking Prednisone, Plaquenil or Advil; my joint pain is gone, my skin looks great and I feel good. The book explains what works and outlines strategies for changing your lifestyle. I know it sounds too good to be true, but it's very true. The information in this book changed my life."

Erica Harzewski, California

"I found your book on the Internet. I downloaded it that day, started on the program that day, and within weeks could tell that symptoms that had never disappeared were now disappearing. After just 3 weeks, I was lupus symptom free with a sed rate of 1 and a CRP-neg. WOW - I feel great!"

Tami Finley, R.N., Texas

"I made changes to my diet a little over a week ago, and have started feeling results already. I have lost most of my muscle and joint pain. I used to feel it all day, now I only feel a little stiff and achy in the morning. Once I am on my morning walk, the stiffness is gone for the rest of the day. Also, the butterfly rash on my face has faded."

Jeanette Karr, Michigan

"I have lupus and am a twenty-six year old mother of three beautiful kids. I have not been able to open their baby food jars or even take them for walks. Everyone suffering from this debilitating disease knows what I am talking about, and I empathize with all of you."

"Just eleven days after starting the diet I can open jars of baby food, and I have so much energy! I am soooo happy!! I played with my children today and I am crying tears of joy right now. This diet worked for me after six months of Cytoxan several different medications and three years of Prednisone with side effects. I am so thrilled to be able to type an email without frequent breaks. Love to all."

Jennie Stansel, Alaska

"I am 76 years old and have lupus. I am amazed how good I feel after just two months of changing my diet. There's a spring in my steps that I haven't had in a long time. Please send three more books for my grown daughters... they said they want to do what I'm doing - because I look so great."

Gwen Usher, Australia

"My results from following your program have been impressive. My joint pain is noticeably improved. As a bonus, my resting heart rate has lowered from 70 to 55, cholesterol from 210 to 150, blood pressure from 140/80 to 100/75 and I've lost about ten unwanted pounds. This is the easiest "diet" I have ever been on, and these results let me know I am on the right track."

Randy Shaull, Indiana

The

Lupus Recovery Diet

A Natural Approach to Autoimmune Disease That Really Works

Jill Harrington

Harbor Point Publishing
Richmond, Virginia

ISBN-10: 0-9758707-1-8
ISBN-13: 978-0-9758707-1-6

Library of Congress Control Number: 2007926173

Harbor Point Publishing, Richmond, VA 23238   USA

Get More Recipes...

Jill wants to share even more of more of her favorite recipes with you. Just go to this special page on her website: www.LupusRecoveryDiet.com/recipes

You'll also see additional updated resources at her website; articles, audio books, cook books, videos, kitchen supplies, and more...

www.LupusRecoveryDiet.com/recipes

Contents

"The human body has one ability not possessed by any other machine—the ability to repair itself."

— George E. Kriley, Jr., MD

"The doctor of the future will give no medication, but will interest his patients in the care of the human frame—in diet and in the cause and prevention of disease."

—Thomas Edison, 1847-1931

The Lupus Recovery Diet

Note to the Reader

This book is not intended to provide medical advice or to be a substitute for medical advice from your personal physician. This information is not intended to diagnose, treat, cure or prevent any disease.

The information provided in this book is intended to describe the potential benefits of a plant based diet and therapeutic fasting. However, any decision involving the treatment of an illness should be made only after consulting the physician of your choice.

Do not start, stop, or change medications without professional medical advice, and do not change your diet if you are ill or on medication, except while under the care of a physician. Neither this nor any other book should be used as a substitute for professional medical advice or treatment.

Neither the author nor the publisher shall be liable or responsible for any loss, injury, or damage caused or alleged to be caused directly or indirectly from any information or suggestion in this book. The statements in the book have not been evaluated by the U.S. Drug and Food Administration.

The Lupus Recovery Diet

Introduction

"One of the most frequently asked questions from patients is whether diet has any role in lupus or rheumatoid arthritis."

—Horst Muller, Balneology and Rehabilitation Sciences Research Institute

Many books have already been written on lupus. Why one more? And why should you read it? I recovered from lupus twelve years ago, using a specific diet and lifestyle. I am not the only one who has done this; other people have experienced the same results. Yet, you've probably been told that diet has nothing to do with lupus and that you have to live with it for the rest of your life.

This book is a compilation of stories of people who have recovered from lupus, rheumatoid arthritis, and fibromyalgia—along with details of the similar dietary program we used, many delicious recipes, and overviews of scientific studies and clinical trials done on the effects of diet on autoimmune disease.

I wrote this book because most of the books already written are about "coping with", "living with", "dealing with", "embracing", and "learning to live with" lupus. Whether you search lupus on the Internet or read the books, the message is all the same...one of doom and gloom. It is depressing to just read about lupus, let alone to have it.

This book is for people who are searching for help with their autoimmune disorder. Some of you already have a diagnosis of lupus or rheumatoid arthritis. Others may have been told they have a "lupus-like" autoimmune disease, but are struggling to get a definite diagnosis.

This diet and lifestyle is something that can help you now, whether you already have a diagnosis of an autoimmune disease or even while you and your doctor are searching for a definite diagnosis.

I wish someone had handed me a book like this fifteen years ago. It would have saved me three years of pain and agony.

An aggressive dietary approach can often be the first method of treatment. There are no negative side effects as with drugs, and the results can be remarkable.

Many people are looking for alternative treatments that work, but the information is not easy to find. This book is a compilation of the resources that I have discovered over the past fourteen years. During my research, I interviewed people who have overcome autoimmune disease and doctors who have experience treating lupus with diet and lifestyle. I hope our stories can reach out to those of you who are searching for help.

After reading the personal success stories, you will see that diet, exercise, sleep, and stress reduction can have a dramatic effect on lupus, rheumatoid arthritis, fibromyalgia and other autoimmune diseases.

The method outlined is not mere theory or guesswork. Incredible as it seems, it has been shown to work consistently and predictably.

Will this diet and lifestyle help everyone overcome lupus? The reversal of the disease becomes less predictable once a body becomes damaged by the long-term use of steroids and immunosuppressive drugs. However, most people will still benefit – even if they do not obtain a full recovery. The earlier in the disease process you start, the easier it is to reverse.

There is little disagreement among health practitioners that eating a healthy diet, getting enough sleep, engaging in moderate exercise and reducing stress are beneficial in the management of the disease of lupus.

What isn't widely known is how much of an effect diet, sleep, and exercise can have in lupus and other autoimmune diseases. The people in this book have found that diet, sleep and exercise can make a *profound* difference.

You'll read about Vanessa, a seventeen year-old girl who had lupus nephritis, with her kidney at a dangerous stage 4. Within three months of making some basic dietary changes, her kidney had dramatic improvement and was close to a normal stage 1.

For years, Debbie's lupus made her so sensitive to the sun that she had to keep all the drapes closed in her house. She now loves being in the sunshine, and is active again with her family in outdoor adventures.

Diane suffered with rheumatoid arthritis, but refused to take Methotrexate because she and her husband desperately wanted to have a baby. Within eighteen-months of starting the program outlined in this book, she was symptom-free and became pregnant. She now has four children, and the health and energy to keep up with them.

While writing this chapter, I spoke with Erica, who has struggled with lupus for five years. She told me that after following this program for the last few months, her knuckles were no longer red and swollen, her eczema and severe dandruff were gone, and that most importantly, she felt overwhelming joy. She didn't realize how down and depressed she had been for so long, and is now amazed by these new feelings of joy. She and her husband are planning a backpacking trip, something she never thought she'd be able to do again.

In this book we have shared our stories so you can see that it's not just an isolated case or two...that many people have regained their health, through diet, moderate exercise, and lots of good, deep sleep.

The stories of recovery in this book are not from "spontaneous remissions", but from a specific diet and lifestyle program. The results have been long lasting.

This book is not about taking drugs or supplements. It's not about coping with or living with lupus. It's how to get lupus out of your life.

Once you have read the personal stories of recovery and you are inspired to create your own success story—the details and resources that can help you make it happen are in this book. I hope to include your success story in the book's next edition.

Part One:
Recovery Stories

"The person who says it cannot be done should not interrupt the person doing it".

—Chinese proverb

MY RECOVERY FROM SYSTEMIC LUPUS

"Most people would never guess that my fingers used to hurt so much that I couldn't hold someone's hand. Now I play tournament tennis."

—Jill Harrington

I was only thirty-two years old, yet I woke up one day with curled and painful fingers that looked like they belonged to an eighty-two year old arthritic woman.

My lupus story began fifteen years ago, in March of 1992. In the previous twelve months I had experienced a great deal of stress; a separation and divorce, loss of a job, sale of a house, new job, a move to a new city, purchase of another house, and a new relationship. I also began commuting an hour and a half each way to work.

That March, I scheduled a routine gynecologist appointment. The doctor suggested that I see a rheumatologist, because of a newly developed red rash on my face, as well as some laboratory blood work that showed possible signs of lupus.

A year earlier, another doctor had done a few blood tests that showed some potential flags for an autoimmune disorder. The symptoms were minimal and I had put the thought out of mind until this doctor suggested more tests.

Minor Aches and Pains

After an exam, the rheumatologist saw no obvious lupus symptoms to be concerned about, though I did have some moderate Raynaud's symptoms in my hands (very white, bloodless looking fingers). I also felt some minor joint pains in my knees and shoulders, which I assumed were from years of playing sports.

The rheumatologist referred me to a dermatologist, who thought that my rash looked more like a skin condition called rosacea. I was prescribed a topical skin ointment, and told to let either doctor know if anything changed.

Two days after the visit to the rheumatologist, I left town on a business trip, and drove for eight hours. At the hotel that night, my hands were very stiff and painful. My fingers began curling up, and I suddenly felt like an old woman with severe arthritis! After a hot shower, my fingers loosened up and I felt better. Again the next morning my hands were noticeably sore, and the pain and stiffness worsened throughout the day.

The joint pain in my hands spread to my shoulders, and continued to worsen over the next couple of weeks. I tried to ignore the pain. A few weeks later, I finally scheduled another appointment with the doctor, because my wrists began to feel as if someone had hit them with a hammer.

After a brief examination, the rheumatologist implied that I was exaggerating the pain because I showed no obvious signs of inflammation. He drew some blood for laboratory tests and suggested I take Naprosyn, a non-prescription anti-inflammatory drug.

I didn't want to take drugs, without knowing what was causing the pain. I called my father, an orthopedic surgeon, and told him what had been recommended. He suggested that for the next week, I take the medication, exercise daily, and eat normally. That seemed like good advice, and I was sure that I would be fine in a week.

After seven days, there was some improvement, but my fingers remained stiff and my wrists stayed painful. Just closing a car door caused me to wince. Always exhausted and in pain, I moved very slowly.

A week later, I went back to the rheumatologist and heard the results of the laboratory tests. Some of the blood work was abnormal: false positive VDRL, mild neutropenia, high sed rate (measures level of inflammation), a low white blood cell count, a positive antinuclear antibody (ANA) and an abnormal nail fold capillaroscpy (which is very sensitive for picking up connective tissue disease).

Combined with the joint pain; rashes on my face, back and thighs; frequent low-grade fevers; and mild Raynaud's phenomenon, I was given a diagnosis of "undifferentiated connective tissue disease". The rheumatologist prescribed a different anti-inflammatory drug, Voltaren, and told me to come back in three weeks.

Finally, a Diagnosis of Lupus

Over the next few months I continued to experience pain and exhaustion. I was tested for HIV a few times, which gave me something else to worry about. I also underwent a spinal tap to "rule out serious disorder"—I assumed that meant the possibility of cancer.

In August, additional blood tests showed a positive double-stranded DNA. This test result showed that my body was producing antibodies directly against the DNA of my own cells. It can mean that the disease is getting serious, and that vital organs (like kidney, heart or lung) are likely to become involved. This is not a good thing. That test, along with the other tests and symptoms, confirmed a diagnosis of lupus.

In August 1992, the doctor wrote in my chart, "Her disease appears to be manifested by neutropenia, arthralgias, rash, false positive VDRL, positive ANA at 1:32 nucleolar pattern, and positive anti-double-stranded DNA antibodies—which is very specific for lupus."

What this means in English, is that I had low white blood count, joint pain, a red face and back rash, and some blood test results that were very specific to lupus. I was diagnosed quickly; some people agonize with pain and suffering for years before getting a diagnosis.

At first I thought a diagnosis was good news, now we could do something about it. Well, the rheumatologist then hit me with the bad news: there is no known cause and no known cure for lupus. He said I would have lupus and be on medication for the rest of my life.

He continued to say that I probably wouldn't die from lupus, but that I might. He also said that I'd probably need to take steroids at some point, which would make my face puffy, lead to kidney failure and ultimately a kidney transplant. He added the hope that new drugs or treatments may be developed by that time.

Well, I believed in the medical system, after all, my father was a doctor, but this scenario sounded unbelievably awful. What demon had taken over my body? I had always been so healthy and active. Because I didn't know what else to do, I decided to take the prescribed drugs—first Voltaren, and when that didn't help, Tolectin.

The anti-inflammatory drugs didn't improve my symptoms or lab results much, so in October the doctor prescribed Plaquenil. I felt a little better, but not much. My face looked sunburned and I still suffered with a constant fever, low energy, stiffness, and joint pain.

In late November of 1992, while out in the yard, I came in contact with some poison oak. Within a few days, my forearm oozed with blisters. Constant itching kept me up all night. Feeling miserable, I begged for drugs to stop this rash that had flared out of control. I was prescribed a five-day dose of Prednisone. Within a few days, I had no more itching AND I had no more joint pain. I was really happy—I thought the lupus was gone!

Learning the Bad News About Medications

I called both my father and the rheumatologist with great excitement. Unfortunately, they explained that Prednisone, a corticosteroid, is a very strong anti-inflammatory drug, which just suppresses the immune system response. At first I thought I had been cured...but then learned that I had no more pain because my immune system was forced into submission and couldn't respond, even though it wanted to.

I thought that maybe I just needed a smarter, more experienced doctor, so in December I sought a second opinion from a rheumatologist at the Medical College of Virginia. The new doctor agreed with everything the first doctor had done, but was easier to talk with, so I continued to see him.

My symptoms were noticeably better, as the Prednisone had knocked out the immune response, and the Plaquenil was keeping it down. However, I still had constant fatigue and stiffness, though I was learning how to live with it. My boyfriend didn't understand anything about lupus, and pretended that nothing was wrong. I learned to just not talk about how bad I felt and tried to keep up with my normal activities.

Determined to Learn

I wanted to know more about the immune system and how it worked. I read everything I could get my hands on about lupus, researching both traditional and alternative treatments and therapies. I tried acupuncture and homeopathic remedies; neither seemed to have any effect on my symptoms.

In October of 1993 I picked up a book that had sat on my shelf since a former boss recommended it a few years earlier. I remembered that it had something to do with health and the importance of what you eat. I found the book, and read about the benefits of eating a lot of fruits and vegetables and cutting back on meat and dairy.

They wrote of the importance of a plant-based diet, sleep, exercise, clean air and water. It seemed to make sense, and I partially implemented some changes.

Eating a plant-based diet was not an easy task—but neither was living with lupus. I lived on the Chesapeake Bay in Virginia with a twenty-five foot fishing boat at the backyard dock. I'm sure there was not another plant eater within fifty miles of where I lived! I began by eating more fruits and vegetables. Over a six-month period, I stopped eating beef, chicken, and pork. I still ate some cheese, seafood and vegetarian junk foods (like bagels, crackers and diet coke).

My symptoms had been much better following that short dose of Prednisone, and I suspected that the Plaquenil wasn't really doing much. I began tapering down the Plaquenil in December of 1993, and by April of 1994 I stopped taking the drug completely.

In June 1994, two months after stopping the drug, the symptoms reappeared with a vengeance and I felt awful. My hair began falling out. After a shower, my long hair would cover the floor of the shower.

I developed a persistent sore throat, and was referred to an ear, nose and throat specialist. He roughly stuck a metal instrument deep into my throat, and arrogantly proclaimed that there was nothing wrong in there. I now know that for me, a sore throat is a sign that I am exhausted, and need more sleep.

I really didn't want to start the drugs again and continued searching for something that would help.

In August of 1994, I felt really bad, and went to see a M.D. who worked with "holistic" medicine. She prescribed a few vitamins and supplements, yoga, and a vegetarian diet. My neck had been so stiff, that I had to turn my whole body to look to the left while driving. After a few sessions of yoga, my neck loosened up considerably. In about three weeks, I did feel much better. I had minimal symptoms for the next few months, though the joint stiffness and fatigue were always there to some degree.

Causes, Not Symptoms

I was intrigued by the idea that a vegetarian diet could help me with lupus, so I wanted to learn more.

In October of 1994 I ordered cassette tapes from alternative health conferences and listened to them daily on my long work commute. The talks about a whole-food, plant-based diet, sleep, exercise, and stress reduction made a lot of sense to me. I didn't know how much of a difference it would make with this serious lupus condition, but would be grateful for any relief.

From these tapes, I learned that symptoms, like fever and joint pain, are indicators that the body is trying to correct something that is wrong. The fever wasn't the problem—that was just my body trying to correct something.

This was when I began to understand that I needed to address *the causes* of my disorder, not suppress the symptoms. Traditional medicine today acknowledges that all they know how to do with lupus is treat and suppress the symptoms.

Listening to these health promotion tapes, I learned about the importance of eating a plant-based, whole-food diet. Speaker after speaker explained the benefits of eating this way, and how the body is able to heal itself once you stop eating things that interfere with the healing process.

After all, the body heals a cut on your finger...as long as it's kept clean and left alone. If you somehow interfere with the healing, like cutting it in the same place again, or pulling the wound open, or getting it dirty – that the finger could become so infected that eventually it would need to be amputated. I was beginning to understand that the same thing happens on the inside of the body, but it's hard to know when or how you are re-injuring yourself and interfering with the body's natural healing process.

I told my doctor what I had read about the connection of food and lupus. He laughed and told me that I could eat anything I wanted to, because food didn't have anything to do with lupus.

Alfalfa sprouts were the only food the doctors told me not to eat—based on a well-publicized study.

I knew that he had no experience with the effects of diet and lupus, so I decided to continue to eat vegetarian and see what happened. I figured that eating plant foods sure couldn't hurt, and there was the possibility that it would help.

Though my diet had improved considerably, there were still major imbalances in my life. I was still commuting long hours to work, and had begun a side business, selling jewelry in the evenings. I wanted to start my own business, so I could work from home and end my commute.

Well, I almost ended my life instead. I stayed with friends in the city, so that I didn't have to commute every day—but spent several evenings each week hosting jewelry shows. I increased the number of shows towards the end of the year to win a bonus trip to Hawaii.

I remember a show at the end of January—when I drove to Washington, DC—over an hour and a half from work, (in the opposite direction of home), to host a show. I could barely stand up to walk across the room. I was in denial about the seriousness of lupus, and that I was going to have to make some big changes to get well.

Downturn

In February of 1995, the lupus returned with a vengeance. I had a major flare after the trip to Hawaii. The joint pains returned, and my fingers became curled and swollen. I couldn't raise my arms above my shoulders, and my throat was extremely sore.

I decided to take drastic action. I felt that I needed a jump-start to get my lupus under control. I was not following the simple, common sense guidelines that I had read about. I ate a vegetarian diet but still ate cheese (one of my favorite foods), diet cola, breads and crackers. Additionally, I still commuted three hours a day, and didn't get enough sleep. I now know how exhausted I really was.

I needed to cool down the joint inflammation and had read about different ways to do this. Strange as it seemed, people had good success reducing inflammation with medically supervised water-only fasting. I decided to try it, even though my family thought I was nuts. You might imagine what my Dad's (the doctor's) initial reaction was. I really didn't know how much it would help me, but I read that it would also clean out my taste buds and make it easier to stop eating junk foods like salt and sugar.

After thinking about it for a few months, I planned a stay at TrueNorth Health, a fasting center in California. I wanted a brand-new start, beginning with a long rest (*never* do a water-only fast without medical supervision).

My Symptoms Vanish!

I went to the TrueNorth Health Center in California, where they conduct medically supervised water fasts. I was in a lot of pain and barely able to walk when I arrived, with a very high sed rate of 98—which indicated a lot of internal inflammation.

Unbelievable as it sounds, all my joint pain completely disappeared within seven days of consuming nothing but purified water. Seven days! This after three years of agony!

At TrueNorth, doctors gave daily talks, and I learned even more about the effects of diet, sleep and exercise on my health. I became a believer in the body's ability to heal itself—I just had to learn to get out and stay out of its way.

I wanted to keep feeling this good, and was now motivated to adhere to a healthful, whole-food vegan diet.

I left the center looking and feeling like a teenager. My face was cool and white for the first time in years—not that glaring, bright red. My joints felt normal and I had so much energy. My taste buds had been reset; and now even simple foods tasted delicious. I lost some excess weight, and looked and felt great.

My Doctor Dismisses My Story

Once back in Virginia, I rushed to visit my rheumatologist, who was on staff at a teaching, university hospital. I just knew that he would be fascinated by my story. When I told him of my experiences and of my newfound health, he listened politely, and then wrote "spontaneous recovery" in my chart.

I was shocked. Spontaneous recovery! You try drinking just water for a week, and tell me how spontaneous it seems. He was not in the least bit interested in hearing the details about my experience.

Keep this in mind when your doctor insists that diet has nothing to do with lupus. It is possible that he or she doesn't listen to patients who tell them that what they eat affects how they feel. The concept is so different than what they were taught in medical school.

My Program

In addition to eating a vegan, whole foods diet, I started sleeping more—nine to ten hours a night. I also walked outside or jumped on a rebounder (a mini-trampoline) every day.

Once my taste buds adjusted to not eating salt and grease, I didn't feel I was giving up any foods; rather, I discovered the great taste of simple whole foods. I've even won a few cooking contests with some of my really simple recipes. I love eating an all plant-based diet.

Today I continue to eat low-fat, vegan, whole-foods. This includes a lot of leafy greens, fresh vegetables, fruits, avocados, and a few nuts and seeds. I also eat potatoes, sweet potatoes, squashes, beans, brown rice and cooked vegetables (see the recipe section for more delicious choices).

On occasions, mainly when socializing or eating out, I eat some foods that contain cooked oil, or processed foods like tofu or breads or crackers...but I never eat any foods that contain animal products. If people comment on my food choices, I just smile and say that I was really sick and that eating this way keeps me feeling great.

Lupus Free for Twelve Years...and Counting!!

Since June of 1995 I have remained free from the symptoms of lupus!

I have experienced other beneficial side benefits as well. Within a few months of changing my diet, my menstrual periods became light with no cramping or pain. After a year or so, I realized that my knees no longer creaked. For many years they had made all sorts of noises when I walked or exercised.

My cholesterol level is about 120 and resting blood pressure fluctuates from 90/60 to 100/70. My bone density measures very high (yes, even without drinking milk or taking calcium supplements). Also, a few years ago I realized that my eyes had become blue! They were blue when I was young, but over the years had become a murky green color.

Today I am very active, and lupus is just not a part of my life. I love all boating and water sports, particularly sailing and kayaking. I play tennis and compete in a U.S. tennis association league. No one who knows me today would ever guess that I used to be in such excruciating pain that I couldn't even hold a tennis racquet, let alone hit an overhead.

I had read about the dietary fundamentals for good health, but didn't realize it would really work for my lupus. Much of the information had been on general health – and not specifically lupus or even autoimmune disease.

I learned that the key was to stop eating foods that cause my immune system to overreact.

I had implemented parts of the message and cut out most animal products. However I didn't really try the program 100%, until I got those immediate results with the fasting. I am not sure that I would have needed to fast if I had initially committed to the food plan, and gotten more sleep and rest. However the fasting experience gave me the belief and motivation I needed to make those changes.

Whether you want to say that my lupus is in remission, asymptomatic, or cured; that it's from the diet and lifestyle or a placebo effect—all I know is that I live without joint pain, fever, exhaustion, and the side effects of toxic drugs. You can call it what you'd like. If this is remission, it's been a twelve-year one— I'll take it—and continue the program that turned my life around.

Please come meet me at: www.LupusRecoveryDiet.com/jill I love to stay in touch with readers, and am constantly posting new information.

Over the years I learned of other people who also successfully controlled their autoimmune disease with this same diet and lifestyle. When I decided to write a book, I wanted to include their stories also. After all, anything can happen to one person.

On the next pages you'll hear from others who also want to share their miraculous experiences with you.

MORE RECOVERY STORIES

VANESSA, *LUPUS NEPHRITIS*

"Now, I am off my medication and can do whatever I want with my life. I thank God for everything."

—Vanessa

"She's so much better! She's like a different person now. We have our Nessa back."

—Shirlene, Vanessa's mother

My name is Vanessa, I live in South Carolina and I'm 19 years old. I was diagnosed with lupus nephritis when I was 17.

I wanted to join the Air Force when I graduated from high school. I had passed all the entrance requirements, even that hard "duck walk". Then they told me that my urine tested too high for protein. So, I drank a lot of water, and tried three more times to pass the test. After the third time and several tests, I was sent to a pediatric nephrologist. My doctor took a look at my lab work and me and said, "You have lupus nephritis and I want to put you into the hospital and do a kidney biopsy tomorrow." Even though I knew this was the next step, I was shocked and scared.

A biopsy was done of my kidney and we found out that it was already in stage 4—which is only one stage away from needing dialysis. I had no other symptoms leading up to this. My face and my feet had been a little swollen, and I had been light headed a few times, but I didn't think much about it.

The next day my doctor did the kidney biopsy. I started taking Lasix, Avapro and Prednisone. In addition, my doctor started me on an aggressive treatment of Cytoxan. This is a really strong monthly intravenous drug that is also used with cancer patients. I had to go to the hospital once a month, stay overnight and have this drug dripped into my veins through a needle. The nurses had to wear biohazardous gloves and be "certified" to handle it. It was really freaky, it made me feel awful.

The plan was for me to take this stuff once a month for the next six months. I would then have another biopsy. If significant improvement were seen, I would then start taking it every other month and then taper off with a biopsy every six months. The doctors said that it would take two years on Cytoxan to get my lupus to go into remission.

I was very disappointed and sad about this diagnosis. All the plans I had, my whole future was changed in an instant. I wanted to go into the Air Force and now I was going to be in a hospital every month instead. I felt labeled, like a diseased outcast.

A friend had suggested that my mom read Dr. John McDougall's book, *McDougall's Medicine: A Challenging Second Opinion*, because my Dad had been taking two blood pressure medications and had just been put on glucophage to try to not get diabetes. As my Mom read Dr. McDougall's explanation of antigens and antigen-antibodies, she realized that it was what the doctor had explained was happening to me. She contacted Dr. McDougall and he encouraged us to try the program in his book.

Mom told my doctor about our plans to start me on the "McDougall Diet." The doctor said that he didn't have a problem with it, and that he had other patients use things like Chinese herbs. My Mom, my Dad and I all started eating a low-fat, vegan diet. I didn't like eating that way—but Mom really wanted me to try it. I didn't want to give up some of my favorite foods, like cheese and pizza, but I was willing to do anything to get off of those drugs. Sometimes I would cry because I was so frustrated and mad.

We ate lots of potatoes, rice, beans, hash browns, pastas, soy products and vegetables. I love A1 sauce and put that on a lot of what I ate. Nut butters are one of my favorite foods. We grind it ourselves. Mom found many good vegan recipes for Thai, Indian and Mexican food. We learned how to go shopping and read every label. I still don't understand how a NON-dairy creamer can have a milk product in it and still be non-dairy. We also found that they sneak whey into everything. We also got some vegan cookbooks and made great soups. I usually ate cold cereal for breakfast and would eat Ramen noodles as soup or a snack, without the chicken flavor of course.

Over the next few months, I stayed overnight in the hospital six times for the Cytoxan treatments. At first we tried the hospital food and asked them to make it vegan. They just don't understand vegan. Mom began packing our food and bringing it with us, because the hospital food was so bad. She always stayed at the hospital with me. I was hooked up to an IV for twenty-five hours, it was really scary.

After I checked in, someone would come and start the IV. They would give me fluids for twelve hours, Cytoxan for one hour, and fluids for another twelve. They gave me the fluid before and after to help protect my kidney from the Cytoxan. It could have made me bleed. They would also do lab work. If they did not get the fluid started early enough, I had to take the Cytoxan in the middle of the night. A certified nurse had to be on duty and sometimes that could be a problem. Often times they wheeled me to a different room, sometimes to a different floor.

Over the next few months, I gained 10 pounds on the Prednisone and my face got all round and puffy looking. I hated what Prednisone did to me. The hair on my face got real dark and I had to wax off a mustache. My hair got fragile and brittle and some of it fell out. I still have lots of stretch marks even though I only gained 10 pounds. They're on my knees, armpits, and all over my hips—just from the Prednisone. I didn't earn them— didn't even get fat for them, and now I have to live with them. My eyes got worse too. I had glasses, but only used them occasionally. Now I have a stronger prescription and have to use them all the time.

I went in for the next kidney biopsy six months later. We asked my doctor if it was possible for my kidney to get down to a category 1, but he said not to get our hopes up too high because that didn't happen too often. He said the kidney usually becomes stable, or gets worse.

When the report came back, instead of getting worse, the kidney had gone from stage 4 disease to almost stage 1! The lab report said, "kidneys show no signs of lupus."

The doctor was amazed—and said that he had never seen that happen before. It was just awesome. He stopped the Cytoxan treatments and began weaning me off of the Prednisone. I continued to take Prednisone for a year, because the doctor was afraid that the lupus would come right back. In his experience, if the labs fluctuate, the lupus is usually flaring again and so he was extra cautious about taking me off the Prednisone.

Everything was fine until the beginning of the following year. Over the holidays there had been lots of sweet treats at the office. I nibbled at some of the foods—and when I went back for the following checkup, my protein level had increased. Mom and I were sure that it was from eating those foods—and asked for a month to straighten things out before increasing the Prednisone. The doctor agreed to give us a month. I strictly followed the diet—and my protein was back down again the following month.

Lupus is so strange and hard to diagnose, because it can attack so many body parts. The scary thing is that kidney disease is silent. It would be easier if I had some noticeable reaction to foods. I don't feel any different—no symptoms—it just shows up as high protein in my urine or my C-3 and C-4 levels changing. So, it's hard to know when something is making it worse.

I really didn't like the food at first—but eventually got used to it, and now I really like how it tastes. It was an obvious choice for me—a life with those nasty drugs or a healthy life eating different foods.

The hardest part is when I'm on the road, hungry, with people who aren't vegan. It's a big hassle. I have to say no I can't eat this, or no I don't eat that. There are some places that I can't even eat. We were at Sam's Club in the food section the other day. Aisle after aisle there was nothing but foods pumped full of chemicals and hidden junk.

Sometimes I think I would like the freedom, the normalcy of being able to eat anything I want. I just want to be normal.

But, I will do ANYTHING to stay off of Prednisone and Cytoxan, so in that way I just love the foods I eat. Some people think it's easier to take a pill than give up all that food. I don't know how someone could take Prednisone, if it does to them what it did to me. They'd rather do that because it's easier? I don't think it's easier, there's no way that I'd want to do that again. Within the first month on Prednisone, my face swelled up to almost double its size. I had to put a smiley face sticker over my face on the family Christmas photo—I looked so gross. I hated the way I looked. Those pictures make me sick.

We even did a juice fast for a week. I felt good while doing it, and really wasn't hungry. Mom always does everything with me. With the juice fast it takes three days to adjust and then it was pretty easy. The first day you are a little bit hungry. On the second day I could tell my body was working on my kidneys because they ached. It really was a good experience. After the third day it was not hard at all. The juice was so good.

I have been medication-free for a year now. They still do a lot of lab work and I have had some small fluctuations in the kidney function tests.

I've recently started eating more whole foods like fruits and vegetables, and less packaged foods. I want to get even healthier, so that I don't have to worry about this coming back. I had quit eating meat and dairy, but up until recently I didn't really eat too many fresh fruits and vegetables.

My parents feel so much better too. My Mom's doctor lowered her thyroid medication and my Dad got off of his blood pressure and diabetes medications.

I'm now going to college and working. I ride my Yamaha V-Star 650 everywhere I go. I'm pretty small and only weigh 100 pounds, so I get a few stares, it's fun. I am in college now majoring in Criminal Justice/Forensics. I want to be a Crime Scene Investigator when I'm done. I love watching Forensic Files and CSI.

My advice to you is to definitely try it. When I first started eating this way I cried, and I thought there was no way that I could do it—because I love food too much. Now, I find that I'm actually becoming a real vegan—and I don't even want to eat meat. Cheese seems nasty—they make it by letting it sit around and age. So it gets a lot easier and it's definitely worth it.

I posted a short version of my story on a bulletin board and a few people wrote and asked me what I had done. I really like helping someone else. People need to know it's possible. I hope that sharing my story will make a big difference in someone's life.

During my first appointment with my Doctor, he said, "she smells like lupus." That was the worst part of the whole thing, I thought he meant that I literally smelled different. After that, I felt terrible. I was no longer the same person I used to be. I was different and could never be the same. They say there is no cure for lupus, and it never goes away. Sometimes I would get so frustrated and cry because I just wanted to be normal. I wanted to be able to eat whatever I want and do whatever I want.

Now, I am off my medication and can do whatever I want with my life. I thank God for everything; if it were not for Him I would not be doing this well. I can't honestly say that I wish I never had lupus. Everything that has happened because of it has made a big difference in who I am, and has made my trust in God much stronger.

Note from Vanessa's Mom, Shirlene

We are so proud of Vanessa. So many people would rather just take a drug and not think about what they eat. We've learned that drugs may make the lab numbers appear normal, but they are not changing the underlying disease.

This whole experience with lupus has been difficult for Vanessa. She feels that it's a life or death situation. She is determined to do what it takes to stay off of those drugs.

All of my kids had some joint pain when they were young; it seemed to be part of growing up. However, Vanessa had more problems than the other kids. My husband and I are retired military, so we took her on post to be tested when she was sixteen. The civilian rheumatologist took several tests. Looking back now, with what I know now, he should have been able to detect the lupus. The general practitioner who referred her to him had even mentioned the possibility of lupus.

Now we keep all of her records. Most doctors want to just keep pumping you with drugs. I noticed that the nephrologist had noted in the chart that "this was an interesting patient."

When Vanessa was first diagnosed, it was pretty scary. Cytoxin can cause bladder cancer and sterility. This was a seventeen-year-old girl we were talking about. At that time we didn't know that we had any choice, so she started on the drugs.

Back then, we didn't realize how bad it was, and that this thing was pretty close to killing her. We had done quite a bit of research on the Internet and were certain that the next step would be to have a kidney biopsy. When the doctor said those words, though, I just felt numb. I could not believe this was happening. I could not believe she was diagnosed with a disease that there is no medical cure for. I felt helpless, afraid and angry. I knew I needed to be strong for Vanessa, but it was hard.

My husband had been taking two blood pressure medications and had been diagnosed with diabetes. When I read Dr. McDougall's book, the descriptions of antigens was what the doctor was saying was happening with Vanessa's body. I contacted Dr. McDougall and he encouraged me to try the program in his book.

I suspected that a change in diet could make a big difference for her. I often felt I was taking things away from her. At times I hated to say, "that is something you shouldn't eat." I almost felt like a villain in her life, snatching away all the "good" things that kids like to eat. I still feel bad at times, like knowing raw nuts are better than cooked ones when we all love peanut butter.

But, now our whole family is enjoying the healthier foods and are continuing to improve our diet even more. I have learned to make great salads. I layer the salad ingredients instead of tossing them. Everything doesn't end up at the bottom then.

We have a great doctor who was willing to work with us on the diet, instead of just saying that it wouldn't help. He would read everything that we brought into him. He has been shocked at the results. He didn't want to take her off of the Prednisone too soon, because lupus can have major flares. We tapered her off over a year's time. Sometimes he is quite skeptical and thinks she will have problems. I can't wait until ten years pass and I can talk to him then about Vanessa's health. He may then admit that the diet worked!

It's heart breaking for a mother to watch her daughter go through this. That last December was the worst. Her face was so bloated; it was the face of a one hundred fifty-pound person, on her one hundred-pound body. She was so sad and hated looking like that.

Many times I cried for her, I wanted to take the disease on me and make her better. I was willing to do anything I could, sacrifice anything to make her well, to keep her off of drugs. To follow the way of traditional medicine is such a hopeless, helpless plan.

It is well worth every sacrifice we have made. She's so much better; she's like a different person now. We have our Nessa back.

DEBBIE, *LUPUS*

"I'm back in the sun, and I have more energy than ever. The Golden Key for me was a small book written in 1922."

—Debbie

I continue to feel like a walking miracle! Not a day goes by without my taking time to appreciate my self-healing body. I just completed my eighth healthy year after living for nineteen years with lupus; a chronic condition which my doctors told me was medically incurable.

When I was in my early thirties I began having health problems that seriously affected my life: fatigue, exhaustion, migraine headaches, rashes, skin lesions, sun sensitivity, hair loss, joint pain, and more. Previous to this I led an active lifestyle with my husband and two young sons, enjoying aerobics, running, swimming and skiing.

Doctors were amazed when they learned of all my symptoms—they said I looked like the picture of health. Examinations and tests proved unsuccessful in determining the cause of the problem. Two years later I saw a dermatologist (my fifth doctor) who diagnosed skin lesions on my scalp as a mild case of psoriasis. When a clump of hair the size of a silver dollar fell from the back of my head, I insisted on a biopsy. The results came back positive for "discoid lupus." The doctor prescribed Prednisone and Plaquenil, and explained that there is no cure nor any known cause for this condition.

After four months I decided to discontinue the medication because of the long-term effects. Staying out of the sun helped me the most, but that was not always possible. So, I applied sunscreen strength 50 daily, wore long sleeves, slacks and a hat outside. I sought to learn about lupus by joining the Lupus

Foundation and reading on my own. Most people with lupus whom I met shared a common hopelessness about the "disease" and agony over the drug treatments.

My search for information led me to a chiropractor trained in nutrition. He encouraged me to give up red meat plus the "four whites": salt, sugar, flour and dairy. He also introduced me to juicing and the principles of food combining. I made these changes and immediately my energy improved, headaches disappeared and other symptoms were lessened. This gave me new determination to find the missing pieces of the puzzle.

The more my body unclogged and cleansed, the better I felt. This motivated me to eat a vegetarian diet and then ultimately my body guided me intuitively to a vegan lifestyle. I found that if I wavered from eating only the good foods my existing symptoms would become worse and past symptoms would return. While I felt much better, the sun still exacerbated my symptoms and the lupus still dictated my activities.

The summer of 1995 was the worst of my life. It was hot, humid and sunny and my symptoms suddenly became more severe than ever. I saw my rheumatologist for a complete work-up. She listened and examined me carefully, but all she could offer was prescription drugs. I went home scared and discouraged. The reality of the situation forced me to evaluate everything I was doing. I decided my system needed more cleansing, not toxic drugs.

That week I decided to exercise more frequently. I began by walking every morning for a half hour or more in the woods. During these walks I gained deeper insight into my health, and it became apparent that exercise helped my body process and remove toxins.

Later in 1995 my son Todd introduced me to the book, "Mucusless Diet Healing System" by Professor Arnold Ehret. It explained the value of eating raw fruits and vegetables for conquering any illness. During the next few months of following Ehret's transitional diet I gained more energy and became symptom-free except for the sun sensitivity. The less cooked food and more raw food I ate, the better I felt, and the more energy I had to resume an active life. I no longer had any doubts that I would be able to conquer the lupus. I was much better, even though the sun sensitivity remained.

During my long ordeal I always drew strength from my loving family's support. I received welcomed words of encouragement and new insights into lupus from other raw food mentors. They offered welcome words of encouragement and new insight into the lupus. They explained that lupus symptoms are nothing more than indications of the body's level of toxemia. I realized that I needed to eat 100% raw food all of the time to allow my body to heal. This understanding gave me new emotional strength. It was time to end this journey with lupus.

I stopped polluting my body with sunscreen and began exposing my bare feet to the early morning sun for five minutes each day, with encouraging results. In mid June 1997 I was feeling well and confident enough to try wearing shorts and a t-shirt. Walking outside, the sun rays hit my legs and gave me the most electrifying sensation of my life! The energy from the sun radiated throughout my body. From that feeling I knew I had conquered the lupus!

Today I continue to eat 100% raw fruits and vegetables and work at balancing and simplifying my life. Learning of "the 100% raw food solution" not only helped give me my life back, it has also given me a natural mind-body-spirit connection that is beyond description. At age fifty-eight I live a healthy and energetic lifestyle! I swim, bicycle, hike, and roller blade with my family— in the sun! I live each new day more joyfully.

The lifestyle I follow today is very simple. I wake early in the morning and drink two glasses of distilled water, with a little lemon or orange to liven it. I then walk in the sun and fresh air. Breakfast is usually fresh, ripe fruit. I'll eat a few raw nuts if I am really hungry, or make a juice from leafy greens if I am feeling stressed (the green juice is very calming).

For lunch or dinner, I'll eat a green salad, raw soup with lots of sea vegetables, greens and veggies or burritos made from sheets of nori (seaweed), nut butters, seeds, or avocado. Sometimes I will blend whatever vegetables are in the fridge, along with an apple and some nuts to make a great dip. I'll spread this on lettuce or cabbage leaves and top it with salsa, avocado and sprouts. I eat a lot of papaya, figs, and berries.

My husband also eats all living food. Before he changed to this way of eating, he was advised to have back surgery. A few years later, at the young age of sixty he entered a triathlon and placed first in his age class, also beating the times of many younger contestants. He continues to cycle, ski, roller blade and play softball—all the things his doctor told him he would probably not be able to do.

The laws of nature have never been complicated or difficult. Food processed into cans, boxes and aluminum trays and laced with untested chemicals are not a natural part of nature. It's when we go outside the realm of those boundaries that get us into trouble.

After my experience with lupus and health issues in our immediate family, our attitude is to only do invasive procedures and drugs as the very last resort.

What I did thirteen years ago is a simple thing to try. Give up meat and the four whites. Hydrate your body with water and fresh made juices. Rest more and exercise in the morning and intuitively your body will guide you to great health. Learn to listen to your body.

When we're invited to someone's house we offer to bring a green salad, fruit salad or make a simple recipe from our favorite living food recipe books, like fettucine alfredo or marinara sauce with angel hair pasta (all raw and delicious). Everyone loves the food we prepare. Friends always tell us they feel better when they eat with us.

None of this information is new. Prof Arnold Ehret wrote his book in the early 1900's. There are many new updated books, information and support online. There are living food potluck suppers across the country. All of this and great health is just waiting for you. So instead of getting up in the morning and wondering how you will get through the day, take your first step toward experiencing how wonderful it feels when life takes less effort and each day becomes the best day ever.

BERYL, *SYSTEMIC LUPUS*

"My skin is so smooth—all those marks from the lupus are gone. People can't believe that I am fifty-eight years old."

—Beryl

I woke up one morning in January of 1995 with severe wrist pain. Over the next few days, the pain worsened and I went to the doctor. They did lots of tests, but didn't know what was wrong with me.

I am from England, but my son lives in New Jersey, and I was living there at the time. It took two years, and many tests, for the doctors to come up with a diagnosis of lupus. During that time, I had also become sensitive to the sun, with a rash across my nose that looked like a butterfly. Severe chest pains forced me to the emergency room on several occasions.

I had upper and lower G.I. tests. I was put on a course of medication, which made me so ill. I was going to the doctor every day. As I said, they did every test they could think of and found nothing. The doctor even told me there was nothing wrong with me and that it was all in my head. They thought I was a hypochondriac!

I was so sick that I lost my appetite. I took a lot of time off from work, so my employer suggested I change my doctor. I followed this advice and found a doctor who told me not to worry and that we would get to the bottom of this. Again I went for more tests, but nothing was found.

I had a special procedure at Morristown General Hospital where they inserted a tube in my throat (it's called an endoscopy), which took pictures of my insides. It came back that I had too much acid in my stomach.

In September of 1997 I woke up one morning and my fingers were so swollen that I couldn't bend them. I went back to my original doctor and had a blood test done. He called me two days later at work to say that they knew what the problem was. He sent me to a rheumatologist. The rheumatologist told me that it took so long for them to find out that I had lupus because it mimics other diseases.

That time was so frustrating. I imagined that I had all kinds of life threatening diseases. I actually was quite relieved when they finally said it was lupus.

I started taking Predisone and Plaquenil. The steroids helped with the joint pain, but I went from a size eight dress to a size fourteen! Not too long after that, I found out that the steroids had also caused me to develop diabetes.

In December 1997, I was also diagnosed with a brain tumor, and I had surgery the following month. My sister came from London to be with me. She stayed for two weeks after my surgery. Both my parents passed away in October 1998, my Father on the 2nd and my Mum on the 4th. I was devastated! Since my boys had grown up, my sisters suggested I come back to England.

I wasn't ready to move. I went back to work for a few months, then terminated my job in November 1999 and went back to London in December 1999. I was unstable on my feet, and was unable to travel on my own, so my sister came back to the US to accompany me back to London. It was a very emotional and frustrating time.

In June of 2000, once back in England, my church sponsored a program on natural health remedies. It was a three-day seminar, and sixty people attended. It was put on by Calvin Thrash and Uchee Pines, a non-profit health education organization from the United States.

The seminar was about four hours each day; the material presented was very interesting. They said if you were suffering from any autoimmune disease they could help you get better and get off drugs, even if you had been on them for a long time.

They also mentioned how you could get off the drugs by eating the right kinds of food, exercising and by your lifestyle. This appealed to me very much and I really wanted to get off these drugs as they were ruining my life and I was very depressed. They also spoke about the poison you get from chemotherapy and radiation. Lots of people go to Uchee Pines after cancer surgery.

I found it amusing that I had to come all the way back to England to learn about an organization that wasn't too far from where I had been living in the States!

In 2000, I went to the US to attend a two-week program at Uchee Pines. They are in Alabama, close to Columbia, GA. I arrived with a butterfly rash on my nose, and limping with a lot of joint pain.

I loved it so much there. We ate an all vegan diet and the food was very good. We had massages and "hot and cold" treatments—alternating between hot baths and cold showers. They are so invigorating.

While there, I was gradually weaned off my medication for the diabetes. The steroid medication was also lowered, and I weaned off of the steroids over a four-month period.

Sometimes when I tell people that I eat a vegan diet, they are amazed and ask what I supplement the fruits and vegetables with. I explain all the different foods I eat, and how delicious they are.

I have been off of all medications since 2000. I am a total vegan and drink fresh juices every day. I don't eat fried foods anymore. Now I eat baked, steamed or roasted dishes with little or no oil and no animal products. Some of my favorite foods are cheeseless pizza, lasagna and interesting salads.

I attended Uchee Pines again in 2002. I felt I needed a tune up. I just love being there. The doctors and staff at Uchee Pines are wonderful people. I am sure that God sent them to help others, they are very special people. Uchee Pines is run by Seventh Day Adventists, but all faiths and denominations are welcome there. Religion is not preached to the guests, though the power of prayer is strong.

I know that the program and my new lifestyle helped me recover from lupus, but first and foremost I feel it is my strong belief in God, my Creator.

Now, at home, every week I go a local spa in London where I do a hot sauna, then a cold shower, and then back to the Jacuzzi. This helps my body get rid of built-up poisons. For exercise, I usually go to the gym and I do a lot of walking around the city.

I have blood work done every three months, and the lupus is totally under control. The rheumatologist doesn't know that I'm not taking the medications. I decided not to tell them, as I didn't want to argue about it.

My skin is so smooth—all those marks from the lupus are gone. People can't believe that I am fifty-eight years old.

I am still concerned that the brain tumor may return. I continue to work on my health, and only wish that I had known years ago what I know now.

DEBORAH, *DISCOID LUPUS*

"I felt that disease within my body had power over me. Now I am free."

— Deborah

I overcame discoid lupus within six weeks.

I am a former nurse and am now a massage therapist. I really like my work and meet many interesting people. Little did I know how that would eventually help me regain my health.

Two years ago I developed a rash on my face and in my scalp. I went to a dermatologist, and was diagnosed with a skin condition called discoid lupus. The doctor said there was no cure for this condition, and that my skin could become very inflamed and develop heavy scarring. She prescribed a medication that I was supposed to take for seven months.

After thinking about it, I decided that I would rather try something else first. For years, I had done some massage work for the patients of Dr. Joel Fuhrman. In addition to his regular practice, he also ran a fasting clinic. As a visiting masseuse, I talked to people who fasted, and they said that their stiffness and pain had gone away. I noticed that their skin was often soft and beautiful during fasting. I decided to call Dr. Fuhrman, before taking any drugs.

He recommended that I eat a plant-based diet, with a lot of green vegetables for six weeks. I ate lots of spinach, kale and broccoli. Sometimes I ate it raw, blended with an apple, and sometimes I ate it steamed. I also ate beans and salad, and a few cooked starchy vegetables. I loved eating green pea pods, dipped in avocado. I also ate ground flax seed, omega 3 oil, and a multivitamin.

The first week, I felt like there was a sunburn on the inside of my body—it was freaky. On the sixth day, I felt really warm and my skin felt like it was crawling. I called my doctor in a panic. He said that what was happening was really good, that my skin cells were reacting and healing. With his encouragement, I continued, and in five more days, I felt great! The stiffness, pain and rash had gone away. I continued to eat this way for another four weeks.

There were lots of benefits. I lost seventeen pounds, that I wanted to lose. My skin became radiant, and people were asking what I had done to myself. I often heard, "you look wonderful." People would even stop me on the street and ask about my skin. All that chlorophyll from the green plants was so good for it.

The diet was easy for me to follow. I was not hungry. People would ask where I was getting my protein and some thought it a bit unusual when I explained that I got it from broccoli and spinach.

The empowerment I found with getting rid of the lupus helped me in all areas of my life.

I stayed on the mostly green plant diet from April to September. I don't always eat that way anymore. I don't have any more problems with my skin. I did notice that when I started eating sugar and wheat, my skin lost that radiance.

If I eat too much sugar or don't eat enough greens, I can start to feel stiff again. If I am not careful and eat much fish or chicken, I get little bumps on my skin. I've learned that if I go back to a plant based diet and drink lots of water, the bumps go away.

I was really proud of the results I had gotten. I went back to the dermatologist to share my experience with her. She got irate and told me that it was ridiculous nonsense, and that I was stupid to not take the medicine. She then said that she didn't want to work with me anymore, and ordered me out of her office. I was so upset. I thought she'd be happy to hear my news, and instead she screamed at me and told me I was stupid.

Many medical doctors are so entrenched in the whys and wherefores—if it's not medical based, they don't want to believe it. I was lucky that I found someone who could teach me the power of the foods I eat.

I used to feel that the disease within my body had power over me. Now I am free.

DAVE, *SARCOIDOSIS, DIABETES, LUPUS*

"The doctors at the Veteran's Administration Hospital were stunned...He and the other doctors didn't believe me when I told them that I had stopped taking insulin and my blood sugars were perfectly normal, they had never seen anyone reverse and get off insulin."

— Dave

I have always been a lighthearted, fun-loving and optimistic individual. My mom told me that when I was a baby I never cried, I just smiled all the time. The same is true today, everyone is always commenting on the fact that I smile all the time. Even when I was faced with extreme health challenges, I was able to maintain my youthful optimism, which I am convinced helped me overcome what seemed like a hopeless situation.

I got out of the Army in 1997, at the age of thirty-three, in fact, I got out on my birthday, talk about a birthday present. I had been a paratrooper and enjoyed physically competing with guys ten to twelve years younger than myself. During my exit appointment at the Veterans Hospital in Charlotte, North Carolina, I was told that I would eventually develop arthritis in my neck, back, knees and ankles.

After getting out of the Army, I moved to America's Finest City, San Diego, California, to resume my career as an architect. I always thought that I wouldn't have to worry about the arthritis until much later in life. However, by the time I turned thirty-five, I had begun to feel joint pain in my knees and fingers.

In early spring, 1999, I noticed a lump on the side of my neck. My doctor told me that it was probably just a swollen salivary gland and I should not worry about it. By summer, I became ill and was diagnosed with the flu. My doctor told me that it had nothing at all to do with the lump on my neck. My doctor gave me antibiotics and the flu cleared up. A month later I got sick again and was diagnosed with a sinus infection and given antibiotics again. For the rest of the year, I got sick every month, and every month I was told that I had either a sinus infection or the flu and was given antibiotics.

This went on until Christmas Eve of that year, when at our family's Christmas dinner, my nose suddenly started to run as though someone had turned on a faucet (yuck). It was really quite a sight; my nose ran for several hours before stopping. Once again, I was told that I had a sinus infection and that it had nothing at all to do with the lump on my neck.

Starting in January of 2000, I began throwing up every morning. I would have thought that I was pregnant, if that weren't biologically impossible. By the end of January, I was throwing up three to four times an hour. I was not the most popular person at work during this time as the walls in the bathroom are covered with tile and the sound of me barfing echoed quite loudly. I was very afraid of losing my job since I was grossing out most of my co-workers.

I had gone to several doctors and emergency rooms, and was always diagnosed with the flu, and given antibiotics. The antibiotics no longer worked for me as I continued to throw up daily for over two months, and by this time a second lump appeared on my neck. Two different emergency room doctors turned me away and told me to go home and take some aspirin.

As a last resort, I went to the Veteran's Administration Hospital. They quickly determined that I was really sick and first thought it was either AIDS or lung cancer. I had a multitude of appointments with several VA doctors over the next few weeks. Each time I saw one of the doctors, they would begin by telling me that this was a very serious situation. It wasn't what the doctors were telling me that bothered me, it was the tone of voice that they used, they spoke very solemnly as they reiterated the seriousness of my condition.

Finally, after much testing, they determined that I had a lung infection and sarcoidosis, a rare autoimmune disease, usually manifested in African American and Scandinavian women. Figure that one out! Pulmonary sarcoidosis is an autoimmune disease involving the lungs; I had lost over fifty percent of my lung capacity. They began treating me with high doses of Prednisone.

Before prescribing the Prednisone, my doctor warned me of a few side effects: weight gain, a feeling of euphoria and a hunchback. I figured that anything was better than throwing up, so I quickly agreed to take the Prednisone. By the next morning, I had stopped throwing up and the lumps in my neck were significantly smaller than they had been. The day after that, the lumps were completely gone, I was ecstatic. I also immediately found out what the doctor meant by feeling euphoric. I had so much energy that I felt like a hyperactive child, I couldn't sit still. I had so much energy that I could not sleep at night.

I would wake up very early, go to the 24-hour gym for an hour and a half, go for a walk for several miles, and still make it in to the office before 6 am, most of the time I would get there before 5 am. Needless to say, my boss was delighted that I would get there so early. At lunch, I would go for another long walk, and as soon as I got off from work, I went straight to the gym again. I would go for another walk late in the evening just to tire myself out so that I could go to bed and get some sleep. No matter what time I went to bed, I always seemed to wake up at 1am, fully alert and unable to go back to sleep, and feeling so energetic that I couldn't lie there any more.

When the doctor told me that I would gain some weight while taking Prednisone, I was thinking that I would gain maybe five or ten pounds. I actually consistently gained between ten to twelve pounds a month until I ballooned up to three hundred sixty-four pounds. Even with all of the exercise I was doing, I still gained weight. That Prednisone is dangerous stuff.

Fortunately, I did not get the hump in my back, I had been afraid that I would turn into the hunchback of San Diego when my doctor warned me of that particular side effect. What my doctor did not warn me about though, was that Prednisone could cause very vivid dreams. Holy cow, did I have some wild and weird dreams at night! When I told people about the weird dreams I was having, one of my friends told everyone that my place was haunted and I was possessed. Hey, you can always count on your friends for encouragement.

What can I say, regardless of the immense weight gain, lack of sleep, and the never ending cinematic marathon of weird dreams, I was ever so thankful for the Prednisone. However, there was another side effect that my doctor didn't warn me about. By the end of October 2001, I noticed that I had to go talk to Mother Nature (i.e. go to the bathroom) every hour and my vision became blurry.

By mid December, I had to go talk to mother nature several times an hour, and I would get so insatiably thirsty. On Christmas Eve 2001, while visiting my parents in Texas, I was hospitalized with a blood sugar level of 1300, and I was told that I had diabetes (normal blood sugar is 75-100). I began taking 80 units of insulin daily, which was quickly increased to 120 units daily.

Because the diabetes was out of control, the doctors decided to lower the amount of Prednisone that I was taking. By the middle of the summer, 2002, I was down to 4 mg of Prednisone. I had lost a lot of weight without changing my diet, and the diabetes was more controllable.

But then, I quickly developed pain in my knees and fingers, lesions on the back of my legs, a butterfly rash on my face and indescribable fatigue. The doctors said that I had developed lupus. My doctor immediately put me back on 60 mg of prednisone.

Since the VA doctors were the ones to diagnose me when I first got sick, I made the VA my primary care physician. I was now seeing four doctors at the VA—one for the sarcoidois, one for diabetes, one for arthritis and now another one for lupus.

The architectural firm that I work for specializes in forensic architecture among other types of architectural work. In the field of forensics, we investigate building failures and construction defects, and testify in deposition and in court as to what the causes are. When we see major problems and failures of building systems, we are eager to find out what went wrong and try to figure out ways to fix it. Likewise, every time I saw a new doctor, they seemed fascinated with my health since there were so many things wrong with me.

During the summer and fall of 2002, with the increased dosage of Prednisone, the diabetes raged out of control again. I was now up to 170 units of insulin a day and still had blood sugar readings over 300 in the morning and 500 at night. I would wake up every night with severe cramps in my legs that would sometimes take up to fifteen minutes to work the cramps out. My blood pressure was getting quite high, dangerously high for a diabetic; I still had the rash on my face, lesions on my legs, joint pain, and blurry vision. I didn't need a doctor to tell me that my health was becoming critical.

I felt that I had to find an alternative to the Prednisone, since it produced so many really bad side effects. Out of the blue, I received an e-mail from a friend of mine in Florida. The e-mail mentioned a three-day seminar to be held in Southern California, called "Reversing Diabetes and Obesity Naturally."

I looked at the web site and immediately signed up for the seminar. I didn't really think that diabetes could be reversed; I only went there to find out if anyone there knew of an alternative to Prednisone. My health seemed to be spiraling downward fast.

Without the Prednisone the sarcoidosis and other ailments would rage out of control, but with the Prednisone I gained weight and the diabetes flared way out of control, it was the proverbial Catch-22. It seemed that if the sarcoidosis and lupus didn't kill me, the Prednisone would. At this time, the arthritis in my knees and fingers was really beginning to bother me and made it very difficult to walk up stairs, which I often have to do as part of my work.

I couldn't wait to go to the Reversing Diabetes Seminar, I was so eager to go because I just knew that I would find a natural alternative to Prednisone. I counted the days like a child counts the days until Christmas; I had to wait for a month for the seminar, which seemed like an eternity.

From reading the information on the web site, I knew that the Reversing Diabetes program centered around a vegan diet, but I just didn't think about it that much. To be honest though, on my way to the seminar I stopped by Carl's Jr. for a hamburger because I knew I wouldn't be able to eat any meat during the three day program.

The Reversing Diabetes Seminar that was put on by a non-profit organization called The Weimar Institute, based in Weimar, California. The speakers were doctors and health care practitioners who spoke on the health benefits of a plant-based diet and other lifestyle factors, mainly exercise.

We stayed at a resort for the three days and were fed totally vegan meals, which to my surprise, tasted very good. I politely listened to the talks, not believing that the diabetes could be reversed. I figured that I would always be a diabetic, and I figured that as long as I was on Prednisone the diabetes would rage out of control with no way to stop it.

There were many doctors and nurses attending the seminar also, and at each break, I would approach them and ask them about herbal alternatives to Prednisone. I was very discouraged to find out that none of the doctors knew of any.

The seminar started on a Saturday evening and went through Monday evening. When I took my blood sugar reading on Sunday morning, it was 269, quite low compared to what it normally was. I thought it was very strange, but then forgot about it. I woke up that Monday morning and realized that this was the first night in a long time that I had not woken up in the middle of the night with muscle cramps and without having to go to the bathroom at least once an hour.

I was shocked when I took my blood sugar reading and it was 84. I took the reading 2 more times—and each time it was 84. I was ecstatic and literally screamed with excitement; I just couldn't believe it, especially since I was still taking 40 mg of Prednisone a day. I was so excited that I couldn't wait to get back to the seminar and tell everyone.

When I left the seminar on Monday evening, I noticed something very strange as I entered onto the road. It dawned on me that my vision had become perfectly clear. I could read street signs and billboards again; it was like being able to see for the very first time. I was so excited!

So, I decided to continue the diet and lifestyle of the program. My knees were still hurting badly and walking was very difficult. I began walking every day. I live a mile and a half from the beach, and even though it was very painful, I slowly made it to the beach and back.

I started eating all fruit and vegetable meals, with no added animal foods, oils, sugar or white flour. Within three weeks, I was able to stop taking insulin altogether, and my blood sugar level was totally normal. One morning, exactly three weeks after the seminar, I woke up and the pain in my knees and fingers was completely gone.

All of my friends and the people I work with noticed an immediate change in my health. So many of them came up to me and said, "Dave, you have your color back." I felt so much more energetic and within several months I had lost sixty-four pounds. All my friends and family members noticed a big change in my health and all commented on how much better I looked and acted.

As you might imagine, the doctors at the VA Hospital were stunned. The diabetes doctor kept asking me how much insulin I was taking. He and the other doctors didn't believe me when I told them that I had stopped taking insulin and my blood sugars were perfectly normal, they had never seen anyone reverse and get off of insulin. The doctors then gave me Methotrexate in an effort to reduce the dose of Prednisone.

I still had extreme coldness in my toes and feet, which then became numb up to my knees. My toes and even parts of my feet began to turn black. I was now down to 10 mg of Prednisone and I stopped taking the Methotrexate on my own since I felt so much better. In June of 2003, I decided that I wanted to get better even faster, and enrolled in the eighteen-day NEWSTART® program offered by The Weimer Institute.

NEWSTART® was a great experience. There were twenty of us in this session. We were encouraged to get lots of sleep, walk the outdoor trails, attend classes held by the doctors, participate in cooking classes, and eat fantastic low-fat, plant-based foods. I also got massages and hydrotherapy sessions every other day or so, boy, talk about feeling totally relaxed. I lost another nineteen pounds during my stay there, and was feeling better than I ever had by the time I left. The feeling had returned to my feet and legs and my blood pressure also came way down.

In some ways, I'm the stereotypical bachelor; I had always been culinarily challenged. Before adopting a plant base diet, I always ate out. The first recipe I learned at the Center was lentil stew. The first time I tried the recipe by myself at home, it looked like oatmeal. I tried it again the next night with a little less water and it turned out like stuffing. I ate a lot of mistakes when I was learning to cook, but I knew that it was going to be good for me in the long run. Now people actually ask me for my recipes!

My lung function improved drastically and my doctor began reducing the Prednisone. The doctors that I had for lupus, arthritis, and diabetes all told me that they didn't need to see me anymore. By the end of July, I stopped taking the Prednisone on my own.

In late September 2003 I started coughing up lung butter again, and my doctor put me back on 40 mg of Prednisone as a precaution, thinking that I was having a flare-up of the sarcoidosis. At the same time, there had been a lot of mold in my apartment caused by a plumbing leak, and I also had cleaned out my parents gutters and found a dead bird in there, so we're really not sure what the cause of the cough was.

My doctors and I tapered off the Prednisone once again, and I became medication free on my (recent) fortieth birthday. Happy birthday to mc!

MICHELE, *RHEUMATOID ARTHRITIS*

"Someone told me that I was just experiencing a placebo effect. I've never heard of a placebo effect lasting eleven years. The effects of food can be subtle... but you do it long enough, and the effects become obvious."

— Michele

I was diagnosed with rheumatoid arthritis (RA) in the autumn of 1992. I was thirty-seven years old and had two small children, two and four years old, and a demanding full time job. The diagnosis came as a shock. No one else in my family had ever had rheumatoid arthritis, and I didn't expect it or know anything about it. The more I learned about it, the more frightened I was that I wouldn't be able to continue to help support and care for my family.

The symptoms started in the previous summer with pain and stiffness in one knee. I went to an orthopedic doctor. By my second visit with him the pain had spread to both knees and my hands. At first the doctor thought that I might have two separate problems, sore knees and carpal tunnel syndrome in my hands. Finally I was referred to a rheumatologist, because the pain and stiffness had spread to so many other joints. Walking and climbing stairs were difficult by then.

The rheumatologist diagnosed me immediately with rheumatoid arthritis. He said, "We've got to consider how we're going to treat you today as well as twenty years from now." That's when it dawned on me how serious this was. I realized that the man was telling me that I had an incurable, crippling disease. I was terribly upset when I left his office that day.

During that initial visit, the doctor suggested that I stop wearing my wedding ring. Surprised, I told him that I didn't want to do that. He casually said "we can just cut it off your finger when we have to," and kept talking as if he had said nothing important. I couldn't get the image of my wedding ring being cut from my crippled fingers out of my mind.

Ironically, about ten years prior to this, an old family doctor had looked at my hands and told me I was likely to have arthritis someday because I had large knuckles. I wonder if I wasn't predisposed to rheumatoid arthritis due to some strange genetic component. I've also read that stress is often a factor in illness, especially chronic illness. I had been under quite a bit of stress, due to a death in the family, and my mother's declining health, just before my symptoms started.

After my diagnosis, I did some research on rheumatoid arthritis and was frightened by what I read. There's no known cause or cure, and the progression is crippling. I saw pictures of people with advanced RA; their hands were swollen and twisted. No wonder the rheumatologist suggested that I remove my ring. I also learned that the medications used to treat RA had some serious side effects. It seemed like the cures weren't much better than the disease itself.

I tried anti-inflammatory drugs first, which helped some, but were upsetting to my stomach. As time went on, my symptoms worsened. The pain, swelling, and stiffness got worse, and spread to almost every joint in my body. At one point it was difficult to open my mouth wide enough to eat because my jaw was so stiff. I couldn't bend my knees at a ninety-degree angle, and they were visibly swollen, red and hot to the touch. By the time winter came, I couldn't lift my foot high enough to step over a curb without pain.

After a few weeks on Voltaren (a non-steroidal anti-inflammatory drug, often called a NSAID), without much improvement, the rheumatologist suggested Methotrexate. This doctor was young and wanted to treat my illness very aggressively, and with the latest drugs. He told me that one of the side effects of Methotrexate was death, which "they take pretty seriously around his office." I guess he was trying to lighten the mood, but I wasn't in a frame of mind to be amused. I was also not very interested in taking a drug that has a potential side effect of death.

I started wondering if diet could influence my arthritis. Maybe I got the idea from the fact that my mother had gout, and there is a recognized link between diet and gout. I asked the doctor, and he just shook his head. Someone gave me a book from the Arthritis Foundation that clearly stated that if anyone tells you that diet has anything to do with arthritis, that person is a quack. The definitive medical advice was that diet had nothing to do with arthritis. But somehow I just couldn't shut my mind to the possibility.

About six years before this all happened, I was experiencing some back pain. I went to see a doctor who wasn't very polite; I'd have to say he had a poor bedside manner. He suggested I was a hypochondriac, at least in part because nothing showed up on an X-ray. If he had just watched me limp down the hall to the X-ray room, he would have learned more than he did by looking at the X-ray. I also wonder if he didn't take me seriously because I was a woman. I don't think he would have talked down to a man the way he did to me. Anyway, his treatment did little to help me, and his attitude actually hurt.

Then I read a book, "The Y's Way to a Healthy Back", about an exercise program specifically for back pain, sponsored by the YMCA. I followed the exercises and it relieved the back pain in a few days. Largely because of that experience, I became open to alternative ways of doing things.

I also had another experience with alternative treatments during one of my pregnancies. I developed a bladder infection, which are common in pregnant women. The obstetrician, an older man who retired not long afterwards, told me to drink cranberry juice. So, instead of taking antibiotics, I drank a lot of cranberry juice, which contains a substance that kills certain types of bacteria. The infection cleared up in a couple of days!

I wanted to try some alternative therapy for my rheumatoid arthritis. I had read that exercise could help, but at the time, I was in so much pain that I didn't think there was much I could do. Fortunately, I decided to try yoga. Not only did it help, it became an enjoyable lifelong practice, and it led me to the information I was looking for.

At the first class, the instructor asked if anyone had any physical limitations. When I told him about the rheumatoid arthritis, he asked if I had tried diet or any holistic treatment. I told him I hadn't but would like to. He introduced me to another student in the class, who told me she had overcome Crohn's disease, which like rheumatoid arthritis, is a disease of the autoimmune system. She gave me the name and number of her doctor, Dr. Fuhrman.

I went to see him in the spring of 1993, and learned about the "leaky gut" syndrome. Leaky gut syndrome occurs when large amino acids leak through the digestive system wall, and the body's immune system attacks these proteins as invaders. It made sense to me. He explained that antibiotics could cause damage to the gut by killing "good" bacteria.

I took antibiotics for a while due to postnatal complications after the birth of my second child. Also, a lifetime of poor eating habits might have made it difficult for my immune system to function properly. Many foods in the typical American diet contain toxins or allergens that we're not even aware of. It taxes the body to have to deal with all that stuff.

I learned that the anti-inflammatory drugs, although they relieved the pain and swelling somewhat, could also damage my digestive tract, which was already not working well. This reinforced my previous impression that the treatments were worse than the disease.

He recommended that I eat an all plant-based diet, with no animal products. It included only those foods most likely to promote good health and that are free of toxins and possible allergens.

I said that I could probably give up meat pretty easily, but would really miss eating fish. Dr. Fuhrman said "When you get better, you can have fish once or twice a week if you want to." *When you get better.* That really got my attention. The other doctor was ready to cut my wedding ring off my finger. This doctor seemed to take it for granted that I would get better, not worse.

I wanted to get better so much, and here was someone who thought I could and would get better. I decided that I would stick with him. The fact that he felt I could recover meant a lot to me. His confidence, and his clear and logical explanations, gave me the motivation to follow his dietary recommendations 100%. I threw myself totally into the program.

For three weeks, I ate almost nothing but brown rice, steamed vegetables, fruit, salad and oatmeal. I ate no wheat, sugar, dairy, soy, nuts, eggs, or fish. I avoided high protein foods, ate nothing fried or oily, and even stopped using salt. Yes, it was a bland diet, but you'd be surprised how good simple foods can taste. I also took some omega 3 oil, glucosamine, and a multivitamin. I began to see results within a week. The pain and swelling began to subside. I was very encouraged and motivated to continue. I sensed that my body would try to heal itself if I met it half way.

At a three-week checkup, my symptoms had dramatically improved. My pain and stiffness were about one third or one quarter as severe as they had been. I could see, as well as feel, that the swelling in my knees had gone down. The nurse commented that I had lost six pounds. For the first time in my life, I didn't care that I had lost weight. I was so excited about my other results. When you're in pain, you don't care about much else.

The diet was not easy to follow at first. Everything I used to eat was full of ingredients that I was supposed to avoid; salt, sugar, oil, flour, and dairy. In suburban New Jersey, at the time, it was hard to find "health" foods. Now we have a Whole Foods supermarket in town, which has made buying healthy food much easier.

After the first three weeks, I gradually began to add more foods to my diet, one at a time. You're supposed to go slowly to see if the new foods cause a reaction. As the weeks and months went by, I started eating more and more "normally" without ill effects, although I never went back completely to my previous way of eating. I found that I could tolerate a lot of foods without ill effects, but some foods definitely caused a reaction. For example, one day I snacked on several handfuls of dry roasted peanuts, and the next day I had a lot of swelling in my knees.

Part of the reason I was so willing to try this plan was that I figured, what are the side effects of eating healthy? Will any doctor tell you that eating healthy is bad for you? Even the rheumatologist, when I told him about my new diet, agreed that vegetarian is the healthiest way to eat. All medications have side effects, but how could this diet hurt me? In other words, what did I have to lose? I also felt that I had some control, that I could do something to help myself instead of sitting around waiting for pills to take effect.

I considered doing a water-only fast. Fasting is a method of treating disease that has been used for years. That strict diet that I was on for the first three weeks had prepared me for a fast by purifying my body first of many of the toxins and poisons that I had been eating.

I was scared of doing a water fast. Fasting is usually done in a clinic, may last one or two weeks or longer, and I would be away from my family and job. Dr. Fuhrman said I could achieve the same results with diet, but that it would take much longer. I often wish that I had done the fast. If I knew then what I know now, I would have.

I continued to take the drug Volatrin for a few months, though we cut down my dosage. My symptoms gradually but steadily lessened, and after about two years, I felt almost completely "cured". I can't say that it's like it never happened, because there is some damage to my joints, particularly in my knees. My knees are not completely back to their pre-arthritis level of flexibility, but I really only notice it when I'm trying to get into certain yoga positions.

I still have some stiffness when I get up in the morning, or after I've been sitting still for a long time. But these are extremely minor problems compared to what could have happened to me. Besides, most people my age (forty-eight) tell me they experience some occasional stiffness. The important thing is that I live a full, productive life, instead of being crippled like I might have been.

I had a mild set back a few years after my original improvement. It was only a mild flareup, but it was enough to concern me. I wasn't going to go through all that pain again if I could help it. I got back on my program.

Pain is a big motivator. Now that I'm no longer in pain I'm not as motivated to eat well, but I try to most of the time. Now I eat a little fish, and occasionally some cheese or yogurt. I drink soymilk instead of cow's milk. When I cook a turkey for the family on Thanksgiving, I taste it, but otherwise I don't eat any meat, and I don't miss it.

I love refined carbohydrates. I am from an Italian family and was raised on pasta. I just try to make sure that most of the bread and pasta that I eat are whole grain. And I eat a lot of salad. You can eat large amounts of vegetables and consume relatively few calories. This diet change was a permanent change in my life. I didn't stay with the same strict diet as in the beginning, but I have continued to be aware of what I eat.

This past winter I had acute bronchitis and a sinus infection, and I took antibiotics. Within a day or two of taking them I had a horrible flare up of rheumatoid arthritis. I continued to take the antibiotics because I was so sick, but I also went back on the original arthritis reversal diet. Once again, the diet quickly calmed down my joint pain, and within two or three days the pain was totally gone.

Now that I've had rheumatoid arthritis, I can pick out other people who have it by the symptoms they're showing. I sometimes try to share my positive experience with these people. I've found some resistance, however.

I knew a woman who worked in another department at my company who had rheumatoid arthritis. One day, I tentatively told her that I had had great success treating my rheumatoid arthritis with diet. She just smiled and didn't respond. I got the impression that she wasn't interested. Now, she's disabled and had to quit working. I'm sorry I didn't try harder to explain it to her.

I recently told another co-worker who has rheumatoid arthritis about my success with diet. She said she was going to stick with her rheumatologist, and continues to take gold salts. She did say, though, that she was willing to try to adjust her diet somewhat. I don't think that's enough, though. I think you have to really eliminate meat and dairy and junk food from your diet to clean out toxins and give your body a chance to heal itself.

One person told me I was experiencing a placebo effect. I've never heard of a placebo effect lasting eleven years. It is so frustrating when people don't believe me. When I experience a flare up, I go back on the diet, and it works. It's not just coincidence.

When people learn that I have rheumatoid arthritis, they sometimes say something like, "Oh, my aunt has that, she's all twisted up," and they start telling me what her fingers look like or some other sad detail. I always stop them, because I don't want to see that picture. I've worked hard at avoiding that fate. I also feel very sorry for the people who couldn't avoid it. I wish they could have had the opportunity I had, and been willing to take advantage of it.

I think that emotion influences health. Once I felt more positive about my illness, it improved. I changed a lot of things at one time: my diet, my lifestyle, and my attitude. I'm sure the change in diet is what had the strongest effect.

My husband was, and continues to be, very supportive. We were both influenced by the hippie days of the 1960's and 1970's; maybe that's why we're so open-minded. He's always supportive of what I do, unconventional or not. He even learned how to steam vegetables, although he hasn't taken up vegetarianism—but I might be able to persuade him yet!

I try to get my whole family to eat healthy. In the early days, I would make separate food for myself when I prepared a meal for the family. Most of the time now, I'll make a meal that will include rice or pasta and vegetables, and salad, and sometimes meat. I don't eat the meat, of course. The whole family will eat some vegetarian meals, and they don't eat nearly as much meat as they used to.

Now that the kids are teenagers, it's hard to control what they eat. They eat junk that they buy at school or at the local deli. Also, we can't keep those cookies and ice cream out of the house—I don't know how that stuff keeps sneaking in! I don't eat a perfectly healthy diet any more, but apparently I did so long enough for my body to heal itself. I still take omega 3 oil, glucosamine, and vitamins.

A healthy diet can be inconvenient since we Americans are spoiled and are used to fast food. After I changed my eating habits, I found that going out to eat could be a challenge. However, you can almost always get a salad. I've found that Chinese and Italian restaurants offer the best vegetarian choices.

Today, my body does me a favor by letting me know when I've been eating poorly. I pay attention to little warning signs like slight stiffness or indigestion.

Ironically, I work for a large pharmaceutical company. I am not against pharmaceutical drugs, I just think that people are too dependent on them, and too quick to take them when there are better ways to regain health. Most drugs only treat symptoms; a change in diet is much more likely to treat the cause of an illness. I feel that there are times that you need certain drugs, that the body can't always heal itself. But I try a natural approach first. I like to say, take a step outside of the box and think differently.

It's been almost twelve years since that doctor advised me to take off my wedding ring before it got stuck on my finger. I didn't take the ring off. I didn't follow most of his other advice, either.

I took an unconventional approach. I took the road less traveled by. I have no regrets about taking that road. And by the way, I can still pull my wedding ring off my finger.

CHERYL, *FIBROMYALGIA*

"I've been pain free for over four years and I no longer have any of the trigger points. I can climb stairs, and my knees are normal. It sure feels good to reverse something that you were told there is no cure for, and couldn't be reversed. I'm totally convinced that it's this lifestyle."

— Cheryl

My husband and I were both diagnosed with chronic fatigue disorder in 1994. We had been under a great deal of stress with an extended family member. The constant worry and stress was just too much for us to handle. My body reacted with total exhaustion. I remember making a family meal and then being too exhausted to eat. I had to go lie down, and was absolutely bone weary. I was glad that my husband and I both felt this same way, because it is hard to describe this feeling of exhaustion to someone who has not experienced it. I learned to live with the constant exhaustion.

Approximately seven years later, there was another very stressful situation that I had to deal with and this time it was too much. I came down with fibromyalgia. I felt like I was eighty years old. Not only was I exhausted, but also I was in constant pain. I couldn't understand what was going on. I went to see a rheumatologist and he pressed many different areas on my body asking if it hurt. I was sensitive in almost every area.

He explained to me that these are called trigger points, and are used to diagnosis a disease called fibromyalgia. He said there was no cure, but that they could provide me with some pain medication. He suggested that I stay away from cold water and to not exercise when I had pain. Well, I was always in pain, and my two favorite activities were swimming in Lake Tahoe (which is very cold water) and kayaking. I wasn't going to give those things up until I had to!

I have a high pain tolerance, and I now know that I probably had fibromyalgia for some time, but chose to push through the pain instead of using drugs.

Some time later, my husband accepted a job with The Weimar Institute, and we moved to their campus. After a few other assignments, I was assigned to work in the customer service department. My job was to talk to people who called in to get information about Weimar's healthy living program, called NEWSTART®.

The program has been taught for twenty-five years. Attendees live on the four hundred and fifty-acre campus for either an eleven or eighteen day program. They are fed a plant-based, low-fat diet and encouraged to walk the many wooded trails. Medical doctors present talks daily on health, there are massage and hydrotherapy treatments, and hands-on cooking classes.

My new employer explained that I would need to go through the three-week program myself, so that I could intelligently discuss it with people. Many of the people who attend the program come to reverse diabetes and high blood pressure.

I thought that sounded like a great idea; eat good food, exercise, and meet people from around the country. It never even occurred to me that it might impact my fibromyalgia—since the rheumatologist had said that there was no cure or effective treatment.

One morning, in the first week of the program, it dawned on me that I had slept the whole night through. For years I would wake up in the middle of the night with severe pain in my hips and shoulders. I'd have to roll over to relieve the pain. That morning, as I was getting dressed, I noticed that there was more range of motion in my knees, and less pain. I talked to the doctors, and told them that I had slept the whole night, and don't feel the pain. They were not surprised, and told me to just keep paying attention to my body and how I felt.

During the program, I learned that when you have fibromyalgia, there is a buildup of toxins in your body. The NEWSTART® program is excellent for detoxing your body. They have hydrotherapy and massage treatments that help with this. I found out that the Russian steam bath is the very best, because you get rid of the toxins when you perspire. They also have a treatment called the contrast shower, where you are sprayed with high volumes of both hot and cold water.

The food here is all plant-based and low-fat. This kind of food helps the lymphatic system to get rid of those toxins faster by getting more oxygen to the tissues, so they can repair.

So a combination of the plant-based food, spa treatments, good sleep, a peaceful environment and lots of walking while breathing in fresh oxygen was so healing. I noticed more and more mobility and less and less pain every day. By the end of the program, I was pain free and this totally amazed me.

I'll say it again, I was amazed. I participated in the program just as a requirement of my job. I didn't participate with any expectation of improvement in my condition, because the rheumatologist had said that there was no cure.

I was on fire with enthusiasm when I went back to my customer service job. They let me speak with people who called and were suffering with fibromyalgia. I would confidently share my story and persuaded many people to come participate in the program.

The hardest thing for people is that there is so much misleading information. I could hear their confusion, they were scared and didn't know what to do. Many thought that this program sounded too good to be true.

Many people with fibromyalgia have gone into a survival mode, and have numbed out on life. They use all of their energy just to cope with everyday activites.

One woman, Ann, recently attended three sessions of the NEWSTART® program. When she came in, she was on twelve medications and two pain patches. She had been sick with fibromyalgia for twenty years. Because of all the medications, her voice was very monotone and she was pretty much out of it. The first week the doctors took her off four of the medications.

She was also diabetic when she came, and insulin was one of the first things to go. Ann said the program was worth it just for that. She also took pills for pain and high blood pressure.

After the first week, she didn't see a difference in the pain. She was a nurse, and didn't want us to touch the pain patches, as she could just barely tolerate the pain with them. By her third program (six weeks), she was off all medications, and even took the pain patches off. Her mind cleared so much. She could still feel a little pain but was now walking two miles a day, and hadn't been able to walk much when she first got there.

Once Ann returned home, her husband saw such a big difference in her that he started eating the same foods with her. It's now been four weeks since she completed the program, and she has built up to a daily three-mile walk. She is still on the diet and off the medications. Ann is ecstatic, and told me that she never believed that this could happen.

Those who attend the program that have been just recently diagnosed with fibromyalgia become completely pain free while they are here. Others take longer to recuperate; after all, it took them years to get sick. Chronic fatigue is a milder form of fibromyalgia, and people with that condition also do well here.

I no longer have any of the trigger points. I can climb stairs, and my knees are normal. It sure feels good to reverse something that you were told that there is no cure for and couldn't be reversed. I'm totally convinced that it's this lifestyle.

I might have been able to do this on my own, with diet and exercise, but I feel that the very best way to do it is to go through the program. You see it; you eat it, you experience it, and you're immersed. Live physicians guide you, and the atmosphere is so restful. Getting out of your routine gives you time to think, and set new priorities. It's a nurturing environment, which also has the latest cutting edge medical information. Your health is worth it. You learn how to continue the program when you go home.

It's a place of peace. There is a different spirit here. The staff is so kind. Everyone extends simple courtesies. There are students on campus. It feels so good, please go and see for yourself. Doctors are here to walk you through the latest cutting edge information and to guide you through the experience.

Understand the value of your health. If we were dealing with finances, and got these kinds of results, people would be standing in line to sign up.

MERLENE, *FIBROMYALGIA*

"If a drug could have made me feel this good, I would have paid anything for it "

— Merlene

For Valentine's Day of 2004, I gave my new husband the gift of a healthy, energetic wife. I had suffered with fibromyalgia for 18 years, and now felt better than I had in many years.

I completed The NEWSTART® program on Feb 12, 2004, and at fifty-three years old, I recovered my health within eighteen-days. This is why I am so excited to share my story with you.

In September of 1985, I lost my first husband, and my fibromyalgia symptoms started shortly thereafter—in 1986. Since the problems were mostly fatigue and pain, my doctors told me I had PMS. I asked them how I could have PMS all month long, but they had no answers. My symptoms continued to worsen.

I could hardly plan anything, since I never knew how I was going to feel, and I'm sure that stress made my symptoms worse. I learned to live with constant pain and exhaustion. I chose not to take any pain medication. I did, however, take an anti-depressant to help me sleep. After the death of my second husband, and the resulting stress, my symptoms really worsened.

The summer of 2003 was a really bad time for me. I slept a minimum of eleven hours, and up to fourteen hours a day. There was constant muscle and tendon pain. It felt like I had a permanent flu; I ached all over.

I decided to see a new doctor. She touched each of the 18 known fibromyalgia tender points, and at each one, I felt extreme pain. You only need pain in 11 of those spots for a diagnosis. So after all those years, I finally had an official diagnosis—fibromyalgia.

I attended a fibromyalgia education class at Kaiser. But the information presented was too vague. I asked if diet had any connection to fibromyalgia but they weren't sure; they said that not much study had been done on that. Through my own trial and error over the years however, I had discovered that diet did matter: sugar and caffeine definitely triggered my symptoms. Kaiser suggested that low impact walking or swimming would help.

In January of 2003, I met a wonderful man at my gym. We started dating the following May, fell in love, and got married in November, 2003. I worried about how my health would affect our relationship, but he was so supportive. He had retired early and said that his main job now was to take care of me.

While at the mall Christmas shopping, I heard someone behind me in line say "for my fibromyalgia..."

I turned and asked the woman if she had fibromyalgia. She smiled and told me her story: She used to be bedridden five days a week and all the doctors could offer was pain medications. Eventually, she found a health recovery program offered by the Weimar Institute. It is an eighteen-day live in program that teaches you how to regain your health. She said that when she arrived she could barely walk, but now walked five miles a day.

Her story sounded too good to be true. Feeling constant pain and fatigue daily, I looked for the program on the Internet, but couldn't find it. I then got caught up in the holiday season, and didn't find the Weimer Institute website until January.

Turns out it is located in Weimar, CA, less than an hour from my home. I called and asked for a tour, and my husband and I drove over that afternoon. A kind and knowledgeable young man showed us around, and we became convinced that this program would really help me. The next program was starting in a week, on January 25th, and I signed up, even though it meant missing my new husband's birthday.

I knew that the program consisted of a plant-based diet, walking, massage, rest and health education. Prior to attending, I thought that the walking would benefit me the most—and I knew that I could do that part.. I didn't see myself eating a plant-based diet 100%. I figured that once I got home, I would modify it. However, I've had no trouble staying with the plan 100%—because it works and I enjoy the food so much.

Prior to the program, I took medications daily, including one for pain, one for sleep, one for depression, several for allergies, high doses of iron for anemia, medications to stimulate my thyroid, and a hormone replacement. While I have eliminated my dependence on the other medications, I still take the hormone replacement and a mild one to help me sleep.

Every staff member genuinely cared for me and the other attendees. I enjoyed frequent hydrotherapy and massage treatments, both of which really helped to relax my muscles. I thought I would need to continue the treatments to maintain how good I felt, but have not found them necessary.

NEWSTART® classes teach great life changing skills. Their doctors showed me how to get and stay healthy, and how to incorporate these changes into my daily life. For example, I learned how to order healthy options in restaurants. My husband and I enjoy eating with friends after church, and didn't want to give that up. If the restaurant offers avocado on the menu, they can make an avocado, lettuce and tomato sandwich on whole wheat bread with a side of fruit instead of greasy french fries.

The participative cooking classes were fun and informative, and I learned so much by actually doing the preparation instead of just watching someone show us.

I successfully completed the program twelve weeks ago, and while I occasionally have some minor fatigue and muscle/tendon pain, I feel so much better now that I can't even compare how I felt then and I how I feel now. I love the results.

I now sleep eight or nine hours a night without constantly waking up, and I get out of bed with lots of energy.

I faced my biggest challenge when I first returned home. I looked in my kitchen cabinets and realized I had so few foods that I would eat. I replaced everything. At first I spent a lot of time in the grocery store reading labels, but now, it's easy and quick to shop because I know what to buy: fruits and vegetables, whole grains, and products with no or low-fat, low salt, no sugar and no added oils.

My husband, a type A personality, used to wake up in the morning long before I got up at 11 a.m. Now, some days I've worked out on the stair master for an hour before he even stirs. I love to walk outside, and only exercise inside if it's bad weather.

I work out with a trainer at the gym again. I had quit seeing him, because I felt too bad to exercise, but now I feel great. The other day he told me that there is no comparison in how I am now and how I used to be. He said it seemed like I used to even talk in slow motion. My health has improved so much that now I step up and down easily on one piece of equipment that I used to have to hold a rail and pull myself up.

I had been so sick and miserable that I was stuck in a vicious cycle. I didn't feel well enough to make healthy food or exercise, which made me even sicker.

When I left The Weimar Institute, my cholesterol was down from 169 to 131. My blood sugar is now normal, but I had been borderline diabetic when I checked in for the program.

My husband has supported me tremendously. He saw how bad I felt, and how good I feel now. He enjoys all the new foods I cook. We eat the same meals at home, though he occasionally orders chicken when we eat out.

In a typical day I eat a serving of five-grain cereal with seeds, nuts and unsweetened soymilk; potatoes with onion and red bell pepper, whole-wheat toast, and some grapefruit for breakfast. We usually eat a late lunch; today we had vegetable enchiladas, brown rice and beans, and a big salad. Dinner will be a delicious vegetable recipe from the NEWSTART® cookbook, plus fruit and salad. Sometimes our meals are more simple—just salad and fruit or baked potatoes and black beans, with salad.

My diet consists of whole plant foods, low salt, no caffeine, and no added oils. I eat two to three fruits a day, five veggies, some beans and/or nuts, and whole grain foods a couple of times a day. I really don't have room for too much more when I eat all of these delicious and healthy foods.

I usually pick Sunday afternoon to plan a partial menu for the week. I decide on several main dishes, and pick a couple of days to make them. It's been pretty simple.

I stopped eating sugar and caffeine and salt. I struggled to give up the decaffeinated coffee and iced tea. My husband still drinks it, and the smell tempts me a bit—but I just remind myself how good I feel without it.

I stay in touch now with the woman who introduced me to the program, and she suggested keeping these foods on hand: avocados, potatoes, beans—fresh cooked or canned, salad, fresh veggies, and fruit. She said I would always able to make something tasty and satisfying to eat with those basic ingredients. Her husband and kids are not vegan, and she just adds additional ingredients to alter what she makes for herself (like adding ground beef to vegetarian chili).

When people ask me how I can eat like this, I tell them that it's not a diet; it's a way of life. I feel so good, I'd be nuts to eat any other way! When asked about protein, I tell them that the doctors at Weimar explained that we only need about 10% of our calories from protein. It's easy to get enough protein from plant foods. Most people eat way too much protein, which is hard on your body.

Seventeen people attended class with me and everyone enjoyed dramatic improvements in their health. A thirteen-year-old girl with type 1 diabetes was totally insulin and medication free at the end of the session. Many of the other folks were there because they struggled with high cholesterol and weight gain, both of which started to cause other problems. A couple of people lost close to twenty pounds during the eighteen-day session, all while eating lots of delicious foods.

This is the best money I have ever spent, and I spent it on myself! If a drug could make someone feel this good, they would pay anything for it!

One of my good friends who had also dealt with fibromyalgia for years, died from complications of pneumonia. I wish that she had attended the program with me and learned how to regain her health. Now she's gone.

While someone can do many aspects of the NEWSTART® program on their own, I think it would have been so much harder for me. By the time I left the campus, I had already been eating healthy for three weeks, and had plenty of sleep, rest, and exercise. The head doctor even gave me his personal email and home phone number when I left, encouraging me to call him anytime with questions. I've never had another doctor do that!

I thank the Lord every day for this gift of health.

ADDITIONAL RECOVERY STORIES THAT INCLUDE WATER-ONLY FASTING

In this section you will read about people who in addition to dietary changes, underwent a *medically supervised* water-only fast.

Water-only fasting should only be done with proper medical supervision.

Do not ever attempt to fast on your own. You need the proper care and attention of a qualified physician, to insure a safe and effective experience.

As you have already read from the previous stories, people have recovered from autoimmune disease without utilizing fasting. **It is not necessary to fast**, and sometimes a person should absolutely not fast—such as when they are on medication.

You will read more about water-only fasting in the "Fasting" chapter. That chapter has a list of doctors experienced in water-only fasting who you can contact for more information.

MARILYN, RHEUMATOID ARTHRITIS

"I took it step by step, and now rheumatoid arthritis and chronic fatigue are out of my life."

—Marilyn

I was like everyone else I knew in the 1960's. There was no consciousness about anything we ate, or drank, or smoked, or ingested... period. I partied with the best of them and then married a man with whom I drank and smoked.

We ate out often, because we traveled a lot, and I didn't know how to cook. Of course, the cocktail hour was always more important than dinner. All my friends drank and smoked too.

I was married to the second largest cattle feeder in Colorado. Meat, and the smell of manure when it rained, was a big part of my life. During those days I noticed that they were injecting cattle with growth hormones to "fatten" them up and also adding things to their feed to increase their weight for the big kill.

One Sunday evening we stopped by the packing plant, which I had never visited before. While waiting for my husband, I sat in the car watching all the cattle standing in a narrow gated alleyway. I remember being bothered that they had to stand up all night in this narrow alleyway and then in the morning would be pushed up this ramp where, once they entered the building they would be shot in the head, and big hooks lifted them to their slaughter.

Cattle get a great look of fear in their eyes when something happens out of the ordinary. If you move too quickly they get a fearful look and move back. I also remember thinking that those cows would die with fear in them and that would somehow be in the meat I ate (along with the hormones and antibiotics they were fed). However, I decided to repress those worries and continued on with my usual lifestyle until I turned thirty.

Between the ages of nineteen and thirty, I had a lot of surgeries...my guess is about twelve, including a laminectomy of my L-5 area and a complete hysterectomy for early cancer of the cervix. This meant a lot of narcotics, pain pills, and anesthesia. I had many unhealthy side effects from all this surgery and the drugs. I started the beginning of over twenty-five years on the drug Premarin.

A lot happened the year I turned thirty, (including a divorce from the cattleman), but what is relevant to this story is that over the following few years I read and educated myself about foods, pesticides, animal fats, etc. and the negative effects that polluted foods can have on the body. This was the beginning of my consciousness about food, my health, and my body...it was a time of change.

I first gave up red meat, coffee, and all other caffeinated drinks, sugar and salt. I used to drink ten to fifteen cups of coffee a day. Do you know there are over nine teaspoons of sugar in a soft drink? I still don't eat these foods today, unless they are an ingredient in restaurant food.

I moved to California and it was during this transition that I stopped smoking and eating dairy products. I had stopped drinking alcohol those days...just herbal teas. It was during this time that my big health issues began.

This was now the late 1970's and early 1980's. First I started losing my hair...a lot of hair. Within a couple of years I was diagnosed with what at the time was called Epstein Barr disease (now called chronic fatigue syndrome). For seven months I was barely able to move myself around. Getting up to use the bathroom was exhausting and one night I went through every cabinet and cupboard for something to kill myself with, but all I could find on the shelves were vitamins.

Most doctors just looked at me like I was crazy when I tried to explain how bad I felt. I had an open-minded nutrition doctor who helped me through some of it, but even she didn't know how to help much.

I would force myself to sit on an exercise bike and push those pedals, even if I could only go around ten times. I felt that I had just had to exercise to get better.

I began a total vegan diet, and sometime during the seventh month I began to feel better—but for the next ten years or so, suddenly I would feel like I passed through an invisible wall and would have to lie down, with no energy at all. It just was amazing that I could feel fine and then go into some totally different mode within seconds. The stress from these episodes kept me off balance. My hair kept falling out; usually for several months and then it would stop for a while.

In the late 1980's I moved to Cincinnati and within a couple of years my joints were painful and some of my fingers became deformed. My thumb became painfully locked in place. I was still having the episodes of utter exhaustion. As a reminder, I was still eating a vegan diet through all this time (however, it was not the low fat, whole foods diet that I eat now). People in Cincinnati thought I was from a different planet. At that time, there were no acupuncturists, very few health food stores, and almost no organic produce—but I never gave in to the difficulties in keeping up with my diet.

Despite this I was diagnosed with rheumatoid arthritis. I continued to have ebbs of low energy, but I exercised on a regular basis at a gym, roller bladed many miles a week, joined a bike club ...just pushed ahead. I finally had to stop biking because my hands hurt too much.

I moved to Santa Fe, NM in 1996 where I fell back in love with the West—and with a man named Ted. It was a lucky match for me because he had a second degree in alternative medicine, and had researched and studied how the body works and what it needs to be healthy. He also had great expertise in detoxing your body, something I had never done. He started me on juicing and I remember the evening that my thumb first moved.

I was at the gym and it just moved after two years of being locked in place. I kept up the juicing and within a couple of months had total movement back in my thumb area.

I still had a lot of pain in my joints, could hardly move in the mornings and some days needed help getting out of bed because of my back pain. Ted was reading a magazine from the Natural Hygiene Society, and casually mentioned that there were only five fasting clinics left. I didn't respond, because fasting wasn't anything I knew anything about or cared about.

Shortly after, one of my best girlfriends was diagnosed with pancreatic cancer. While I was out of town she went to the Mayo Clinic—where she died. During the drive back from the airport I told Ted that I wanted to go see her, and he told me that she had just died.

I sat in the dark and quietness of the car taking in his news. Then, truly, I heard her say to me, "go do a water fast." I was so shocked because I had never heard of a fasting clinic until two weeks prior and now she just died and I heard her tell me to go do a water fast.

After her funeral I booked myself into the TrueNorth Fasting Center, and that was the beginning of huge leaps in my health. I won't tell you it was fun, because it was not, but amazing things went on with my body. I was terrified at first, but I went back 6 months later for a second fast.

I now fast once a year for ten days, and my rheumatoid arthritis is nowhere to be found. My health has improved so much that I never have those fatigue episodes any longer. Am I in perfect shape? No, but I am also going to be sixty-two this year, something that people never guess by looking at me. Most people never know I used to have rheumatoid arthritis, unless they see the curled ends on a couple of my fingers.

I like to drink fresh juice—and every Saturday I make a juice concoction with all the leftover vegetables. I eat a healthy, whole foods, vegan diet—including lots of fresh fruits and vegetables.

One of my good friends, Karen (whose story is also in this book), began having major problems with rheumatoid arthritis. Ted and I talked with her, and convinced her that she needed to fast. She went to TrueNorth Center and had incredible results. She and I even went to the fasting center together this year.

Considering my past, all the surgeries, all the autoimmune issues, and all the pain and agony, I am full of life and feel very grateful.

KAREN, *RHEUMATOID ARTHRITIS AND FIBROMYALGIA*

"I had gotten so sick that I could not get out of bed by myself. Now I am as active as I ever was."

— Karen

Four years ago, I overcame the ravages of rheumatoid arthritis and fibromyalga. What I did was a bit unconventional, but it worked wonders.

I became a single Mom at age thirty-five, with three kids, ages ten, nine and five years. Suddenly I had to get a job and support the family. I was living in Houston, became a real estate agent, and eventually owned three real estate companies. There was plenty of stress in my life, and I'll admit I ate lunches in my car from fast food restaurants far more than was healthy, because I was constantly on the go.

In my early fifties, around the time I was having premenopausal symptoms, I began to feel terrible. I was excessively tired and weak, and my joints ached. I saw many MD's and eventually ended up being referred to the chief of staff at Texas Research and Rehabilitation Hospital.

When they first diagnosed me with post-polio syndrome, I was in a state of shock and depression. That diagnosis is a really frightening one. The doctor explained that the nerves I had left from having had polio at age 13 were continuing to degenerate. Even though they assured me that I had post polio syndrome, I did not want to believe or accept that diagnosis.

The doctors told me not to do anything physical that I didn't have to do. I was even supposed to use a headset instead of picking up the telephone! This was to save any nerves that I still had left. This was just not anything with which I wanted to be saddled.

Then, about three years ago, my symptoms became much more severe. Eventually, I was diagnosed with rheumatoid arthritis. The rheumatologist told me that fibromyalgia is often a precursor to rheumatoid arthritis. She felt certain rheumatoid arthritis is what I had when I was diagnosed with post-polio syndrome.

The Rheumatologist x-rayed everything on my body and told me that I didn't have any bone or joint damage yet, and that I needed to start taking Methotrexate right away. Although I did not test positive for the rheumatoid arthritis antibody (many people with rheumatoid arthritis do not show the RA factor in blood tests), she was convinced that I was undergoing major damage and must halt it with Methotrexate. My symptoms and other test results led to this diagnosis. I still wonder if that's what I had. Of course, I've since learned that the diagnosis doesn't really matter—what you need to do to recover your health is almost the same regardless of the disorder.

I started swimming four or five days a week and that seemed to help. The only drug I was willing to take was Naprosyn, which is just a little stronger than aspirin. Methotrexate was the next step. I knew people who had lost kidneys and had liver damage after taking Methotrexate.

An alternative practitioner I consulted ran blood tests and told me that I had a "leaky gut". The lab tests showed that I had high levels of animal protein in my blood. These proteins are supposed to stay in your digestive tract. However, when the walls of the digestive tract are damaged, proteins can leak through. I now know that many health care practitioners believe this animal protein leaking into the digestive tract is another cause of RA and other autoimmune diseases.

A good friend of mine, Marilyn, had overcome rheumatoid arthritis. I knew that Marilyn ate some kind of unusual diet, but I didn't realize all the health benefits she received until I began studying and learning about a vegan diet.

My husband and I had lunch with her, and Marilyn's husband, Ted. They explained the concept of natural hygiene, which is basically a diet of plant-based, whole foods. Ted also talked about the importance of the alkaline/acidity level of the body. Using a simple PH revealing paper to test my urine, I discovered that I was very acidic. After just a few days of carrot juicing, I tested much more alkaline. I thought that if a few glasses of fresh juice can cause this healthy change, there must be something to this food and nutrition idea in connection with my health.

Marilyn highly recommended that I start with a water-only fast, as I was so sick. She had fasted the previous year at TrueNorth Health Education Center in Penngrove, CA, and had great results. After talking with Marilyn and reading about fasting, I felt that I had to try it. It seemed I had a choice to make. Either I would try fasting and a diet change or I would take a lethal drug for the rest of my life. I could see no harm, and possibly many healthy benefits, from fasting and a diet change.

When I mentioned diet and fasting to the rheumatologist, she looked at me like "What in the world are you talking about?" I'm not sure what I would have thought of fasting if a good friend hadn't introduced me to it. I was open and looking for something to help me. Timing can be so important in our lives. If I had been diagnosed with RA while living in Houston, I most likely would have taken the drugs, as I would have known of no other option.

I decided to fast in May of 2002, just after being diagnosed with RA. I was at the fasting clinic on Mother's Day. It was frightening at the time, yet I was just as fearful of not trying to heal my own body in this manner. I told Dr. Alan Goldhamer, the Clinic Director, that I was afraid I would go into a hypoglycemic coma and die from not eating protein. He got a good chuckle out of that and said that he'd never had that happen to anyone before and assured me that it wouldn't happen to me.

The ironic thing is that I was diagnosed as hypoglycemic years ago, and doctors told me to eat protein at every meal. If I did not eat enough protein, I became nervous and shaky. I have since learned that eating a diet rich in animal protein spikes blood sugar levels—it's one of the worst things you can do for hypoglycemia. It is highly likely that eating a diet rich in animal protein greatly aggravated my fibromyalga and rheumatoid arthritis. Many physicians greatly underestimate or do not know how diet affects our health. Fortunately, I believe that trend is changing, and more and more doctors are becoming interested in alternative medicine and nutrition.

I wish I had a great story of how my first fast was a breeze and I came home cured of all symptoms. My experience was quite different. I had not prepared for the fast by changing my diet, as I was a bit skeptical about the diet part. The fasting center fed me fresh salad and fruit for three days prior to allowing me to begin the water fast. This helps to clean out the digestive tract, so that while fasting, one does not have intestines full of food.

My fast was a miserable experience. I was hungry at first, but after three days the hunger subsided. The first three days I was emotionally climbing the walls. Then, I had a major flare up and was in excruciating pain. The doctors at the clinic surrounded me with warm heat packs. I was nauseous for the first week or so. It was hard to keep going, but I knew the alternative if this did not work.

The doctors assured me that what I was experiencing was not uncommon for someone as sick as I had been. The good news was that I would have been much more ill while detoxifying from drugs, had I been on them previously. Dr. Goldhamer explained clearly that I would likely have a flare up of RA either during the fast, while I was re-feeding or perhaps both. I must say, he was absolutely correct.

I ended the fast as planned at fourteen days, even though my body would have been better off had I continued for another seven days. I had a nonrefundable airplane ticket, and I had had enough. During the next seven days I stayed at the Center, re-feeding on simple, easy to digest foods. I still felt sick and miserable. When I got home, I mostly stayed in bed. If anything,

I was even more weak than when I left. I honestly felt very depressed that a miraculous cure had not taken place and that I now felt worse than before.

Against most logic, I stuck faithfully to the prescribed diet consisting of whole vegetables, grains and fruit. It occurred to me daily that I had gone through this entire ordeal and not only did not feel better, I felt worse. What was I going to do? What was the rest of my life going to be like?

Two weeks after I came home from TrueNorth, I began feeling stronger. Within ten days, all my joint pain vanished, and for the first time in years, I felt great. Now four years later, I can honestly say I have not had any serious rheumatoid arthritis flair-ups.

Once I was in recovery, I did not return to my rheumatologist—I already knew what he thought. I have shared my experience with my Internist and my Gynecologist. They were happy about the results and have never indicated I was being at all foolish.

I have fallen off the diet. It's easy to do. I eat just a little bit of this and a little bit of that, which leads to a little bit more. Dining out and traveling can make sticking to a strict vegan diet difficult. It's human nature to forget just how badly you had felt, once physical pain and discomfort leaves.

When I do cheat on my diet, I can feel small symptoms within a few days. My feet start getting stiff and get a burning sensation. I can also feel some overall body stiffness. This quickly reminds me to get back on track. It is important to forgive myself, and move on. Once I simplify my diet, those symptoms go away.

I have fasted three times. The second and third time were a "walk in the park" compared to the first experience. Fasting is still not a pleasant experience for me—but I feel so good at the end of it. Many of my friends and family tell me they have never seen me look so rested. I find that consistent with my experience, as I have never felt so rested.

I plan on fasting at the TrueNorth Health Education Center once a year. This last time, Marilyn and I went there at the same time. That made the whole experience much easier and more fun. We spent most of our days talking, sleeping, laughing, reading or lounging in the sun. Doesn't sound all that bad does it?

The readers of this book may wonder how my family has reacted to this new lifestyle. My children are really happy for me—but still consider what I did a bit strange. We don't talk about it much. They had been concerned about me after noticing that I was shuffling my feet and had great difficulty standing up from a sitting position. I think the idea that I could heal myself with diet and fasting has puzzled them.

Converting my husband to a more whole food based diet has been somewhat easy. Gordon had a heart attack several years ago, so changing his eating habits has been good for his health as well as mine. He has been very supportive. When I came home from the first fast, he had a basket of vegetables and flowers on the kitchen counter.

My lifestyle has changed drastically. Just prior to my first fast, in February of 2001, I sold a portion of my real estate business. I cut my work hours from seventy to 20-30 hours a week. I work daily on keeping stress out of my life (that will probably be a life long pursuit)!

I've been able to get back to my gardening and regular workouts. Both had become impossible. I now have enough energy to play with our adorable grandchildren and mostly keep up with a very active husband, who is the great love of my life.

It is my hope that this personal account of my battle, with what could have been a crippling disease, will inspire others facing similar illnesses. There are healthy alternative solutions for recovery of your own good health that need not be dependant upon pharmaceuticals. It has been well worth the journey!

DIANE, *RHEUMATOID ARTHRITIS*

"I refused to take Methotrexate because I wanted to have a baby. Today, I am free of rheumatoid arthritis and have four beautiful children."

— Diane

The story of my illness began about ten years ago, in the spring of 1994. I played indoor tennis for several months, when my wrist began to hurt. I assumed the pain was from the tennis. My thoughts concerning this developing pain in my wrists also centered on my profession. I worked as a consultant for software systems development, and spent many hours working on a computer.

In addition to the stress of my work, my husband and I had also been trying to get pregnant for about six years. In the spring of 1994, I underwent an in vitro procedure. A few days later I became sick as a dog. My health continued to decline over the ensuing weeks.

My ability to work went from fourteen hours a day to not even being able to get out of bed without help from my husband. When I would finally get out of bed and take a shower, I'd have to sleep for a few hours in order to recover my energy. Prior to this time in my life, I had always been very healthy. My husband and I had enjoyed frequent hiking and biking trips as well as many hours of tennis.

Within a few months of this initial 'wrist' pain, my entire body became inflamed. My shoulders, elbows, wrists, hands, knees, ankles and toes were red with inflammation. I could lift my arm only a few inches from my body. It hurt to bend my arm and then flex it straight again. My hand joints were swollen and red, and even the slightest contact with a hard surface would send pain shooting through my entire body. The pain radiating from my hands would take my breath away. Any type of physical effort was exhausting to me. I often found myself bedridden in the afternoons, with a fever of 103 degrees or higher.

By the time I met with my third 'specialist', months after the onslaught of my illness, I was finally diagnosed with rheumatoid arthritis. He insisted that I had to take medication. His analysis of my illness included the expectation that I would be in a wheelchair by the time I was forty-five, and that my lifespan would be reduced by fifteen years. I was thirty-five years old at the time. If I hadn't been in so much pain, I would have gotten up and hit him. I walked out of his office determined that this was not going to be my fate.

Taking drugs was never an option for me. We had been trying to get pregnant for so many years. My infertility doctor informed me that if I started Methatrexate, I would never be able to conceive. Since I wasn't able to accept this outcome, I knew there had to be another answer.

At this point I was desperate for anything that would help me. When you're sick, you're terrified, and you don't know who to listen to. There are so many different approaches to wellness. I'd never been sick a day in my life. I was sick, and did not have a clue what to do for myself.

I had some fear that I was hurting myself by not going to a doctor, but I had already heard what they had to offer. I was out of control of my life. I couldn't work. I seemed to be spending fifteen or more hours a day sleeping. I was losing several pounds a week, and felt very depressed.

During the first summer of my illness, I spent a few months seeing a healing practitioner from my local health food store. He gave me a variety of 'cleansing' teas, massages and advice on changing my diet to a vegetarian diet. This went on for several months, and although I seemed to be enjoying some slight improvements, it was never significant enough to assure me that I was on the right path.

Sometime during the next year, I read an out of print book titled, *Yes, There is a Cure for Arthritis*. The author was a doctor who practiced during the 1960's. He had done extensive research in Europe on natural cures for arthritis. These cures included a vegetarian diet and water fasting. Upon finishing his book, I was convinced that this was the cure for me. The only dilemma was, the clinics and spas mentioned in the book were no longer around.

I finally found a medically supervised fasting clinic, and began my first water fast on Halloween of 1995 and continued until Thanksgiving. I fasted for twenty-one days at the live-in clinic.

There were about ten to twelve other people fasting. We were all fasting for different reasons, but our fascination with food was the same! For many, many hours of each day, we would get together and watch the food channel on TV. Food becomes quite an obsession when you're not eating!

Most of the people in my group did well on their fasts. Some people fasted longer than others, based on their individual illnesses and strength.

Everyone had their own reasons for ending their fast. At the start of the fast, I had rheumatoid arthritis, double pneumonia, constant coughing, a daily fever of 104 degrees, and a sed rate of over 100. My rheumatoid factor had been negative once and positive once, and so I had learned it was not a conclusive indicator of inflammation in my body.

On day three of the fast, I started noticing improvement. My fever and coughing stopped. By day twenty-one of the fast, I could kneel down and put my own socks on. These were major accomplishments!

For the next year and a half, I fasted every six months. Even though I had experienced such good results from the first fast, I was far from being healthy, and my blood work still indicated inflammation in my body.

It took a couple of years for my blood work to get back to normal. My sed rate remained high, close to 80 for a year and a half, even though I felt better. During this period, my body would react almost instantaneously to foods that I could not digest properly. For example, a few times when my husband and I went out to eat, I ordered a plate of pasta with vegetables.

Each time after finishing my meal, I found that I could barely get up from the table unassisted. My joints were inflamed and hurting. It was in this way that I learned the foods that I needed to avoid, in order to feel good.

For a long time this list of 'bad foods' was quite lengthy, and mealtime became quite a chore for me! I ate no processed foods except non-wheat bread, and avoided going out to eat whenever possible. Whenever I had to go somewhere where a meal was being served, I would eat beforehand, since my diet was so restricted.

As my health returned, there was more good news in store. In 1997 I got pregnant! We had been trying to conceive for eight years. I am certain that the fasting got my body healthy enough so that I could conceive. As of this date, we have four beautiful children, three sons and a daughter.

It has now been almost nine years since I first fasted. I have not had joint pain for seven and a half years. My hands still have some deformity in them from the damage that was done early in my illness. The ends of my fingers are bent over. That's the only clue that I was ever sick.

I have been on a mostly vegan diet for the past nine years, which means no dairy, eggs or meat. I eat only non-wheat breads and bake with non-wheat flours. My diet has included a lot of fresh fruits and vegetables, brown rice, sweet potatoes, beans, nuts and soymilk.

Typically, for breakfast, I eat fresh fruit, whole-grain toast and/or a fruit smoothie made with soymilk and fresh fruit. For lunch, I eat salad, soup, hummus or peanut or cashew butter. I also eat fresh fruit in the afternoon. Dinner is usually very simple. I'll eat something like tofu with steamed greens, such as kale, chard or escarole. I also steam a variety of other vegetables and make some brown rice or sweet potato.

I have reactions to all nightshade plants—eggplant, potatoes, onions, tomatoes and peppers. I also react to chocolate, strawberries, blueberries, raspberries and blackberries. So these are excluded from my diet. I recently started eating a little wild, fresh salmon.

As our children have grown, their taste in foods has grown as well. I typically make a kid friendly version of dinner for them, with an adult version for my husband and myself. My husband has only recently come around to this way of eating. For many years I was making three different versions of dinner to feed our growing household. It was quite a bit of work.

At first, it was such a pain to eat differently than everyone else. My attitude now is to "keep it simple" when it comes to food. At first, you're thinking—I have to give up what and what and what? Sometimes I just didn't want to have to work for that meal—it was easier just not to eat! Once the inflammation went away, I was able to eat more variety, and things became easier.

When I first started feeling better, I took my own food to my friends' homes when invited over for dinner—it was so critical for me back then. Now I just ask them to have salad and vegetables and/or pasta and everything will be fine. I usually eat something before I leave the house, so I don't show up hungry and feel tempted by food that I don't want to eat.

What you eat becomes a habit. It's a gradual process—keep in mind that it's just food. It's not like you are going to get up one day and suddenly not eat anything that you're used to eating. It's a "breaking yourself away" process and it takes time. A lot of the motivation for me to stick with this diet came from my healing after the fast.

After my first fast, I could sit down to a meal and if it contained one of the 'forbidden' foods, my body would have an immediate reaction. My joints would become red and swollen within a half hour. It would be painful to walk and every flex of my arm would hurt. It would take about a day of 'good' eating to restore my body to its previous state of wellness.

There are many other ways to get pleasure in life. Food is just one of them, and what good is the temporary pleasure of taste if it causes long-term pain? Maybe the only people that can relate to what I'm saying are those that have experienced the pain of something like rheumatoid arthritis.

I'm finding that more and more people want to eat the way I do. We'll often have people over and I'll fix what I normally eat, and add things like peppers and onions for them. Most people want to lose weight, and really like the food I serve them. I get a lot of satisfaction from cooking for others and my family.

Prior to my first fast, my family was very concerned about me fasting. Friends are still incredulous that I fasted for two weeks. Although, they do admit that it seems to be working. I am in such good health, and am just thriving.

We recently visited a friend of the family, who is a doctor. He said that rheumatoid arthritis never goes away, and that I'm just in remission. I told him it had been a nine-year remission so far, and he was quite surprised. Still, I felt a little discouraged by his response. I just have to remember that I have done something that very few people have done, so not many doctors know about it.

Sleep is another really important factor for me. If I get enough sleep, I can do anything. My success has come from a combination of fasting, eating right and slowing my life down. I used to work so many hours, and was always stressed. Today, life is filled with my children, my husband, family, my continued love for cooking, time to sit and chat with friends and my love and gratitude to God for this wonderful period in my life.

When I was sick, I prayed that when I got better I would be able to share my story with others so that they could get well. Including my story in this book is an answer to my prayers.

If you don't want to fast, even just eating a clean diet is a big step in the right direction. It's an evolutionary process; but doesn't need to be an abrupt change. Begin by eating more fresh, organic fruits and vegetables each day. Preparing whole foods is more work than eating fast foods, but you will begin to plan for your health and make time for yourself in the midst of your busy days.

I believe that this diet is beneficial for anyone, sick or healthy. My children have eaten a vegan diet for the first five years of each of their lives, and have all been extremely healthy. Few, if any ear infections, and precious little of any of the other childhood maladies that most kids get. Even though their diets have changed a bit since they started school, they are still very healthy. My husband, a very healthy guy in his forties, has recently begun eating more of a plant-based diet, and has been dropping pounds that he never thought he would lose!

I hope my story encourages you in your path to wellness Being ill is a scary and lonely place. Listening to conflicting advice from doctors and friends is confusing and frightening. And the thought of not eating for weeks at a time seems ludicrous! But it truly works. I don't believe I am 'special' and that this was a unique experience for me. The doctors who specialize in this have seen it work hundreds of times. My encouragement to you is 'Try it'. You have nothing to lose and everything to gain.

Thanks for reading my story. Please tell a friend or family member who may be living with the awful pain of arthritis. This may be just what they're looking for!

Part Two: The Science

"Science is not an absolute truth in itself, but is really only the search for truth—and only represents the state of our knowledge, or our belief system, at this moment in time."

— Author unknown

WHAT CAUSES LUPUS AND RHEUMATOID ARTHRITIS?

"The cause(s) of lupus is unknown, but there are environmental and genetic factors involved. While scientists believe there is a genetic predisposition to the disease, it is known that environmental factors also play a critical role in triggering lupus."

— Lupus Foundation of America Website

"It is thought that autoimmune diseases, such as lupus, occur when a genetically susceptible individual encounters an unknown environmental agent or trigger. In this circumstance, an abnormal immune response can be initiated that leads to the signs and symptoms of lupus."

— National Institute of Arthritis and Musculosketal Skin Disease

"Faulty genetics loads the gun, lifestyle pulls the trigger."

— Dr. Lamont Murdoch, M.D., Loma Linda University School of Medicine

Researchers do not know what causes lupus or any of the many other autoimmune diseases. There is no known cure. It is commonly thought that a combination of genetic predisposition and environmental factors trigger the disease. The scientific research has primarily focused on the genetic aspects, rather than the environmental.

Some of the environmental factors that are thought to trigger lupus include infections, antibiotics, ultraviolet light, extreme stress, certain drugs, hormones, and certain foods.

Lupus is a very complex disease, but there is a way to stop or slow the activation of the disease process. Stop pulling the trigger. In this book you will learn what some of the major lifestyle and environmental triggers are, and how to avoid them.

The foods you eat are one of the environmental factors that you *can* control.

Since no one knows the cause of lupus, the exact reasons that a low-fat, plant-based diet is effective with lupus are also not scientific fact. However, the connection between the two has been shown repeatedly in research studies, clinical observations and personal experiences.

This chapter provides an overview of some possible reasons that changes in the foods you eat can have such an impact on lupus or rheumatoid arthritis. The second part of this chapter gives details on some of the studies that have shown a connection between the foods you eat and autoimmune disease.

For more detailed explanations of the science, I suggest that you read *Challenging Second Opinion*, chapter 8, by John McDougall, MD and *Fasting and Eating for Health*, chapter 7, by Joel Fuhrman, MD.

First, does it *really* matter to you how diet works, *as long as it does work*?

It's been years since researchers first noted a connection between certain foods and lupus. Since additional studies are slow in coming, you don't need to wait for the results of an elaborate clinical trial. All that really matters is whether or not it can help *you—today*. Try eating this way for yourself, and see how you feel.

The expected side effects are things such as loss of excess weight, lowered cholesterol, lowered blood pressure, and normalized blood sugar levels. Since these side effects can result in lowered risk of heart attack, stroke, and diabetes—there's not much risk to trying a low-fat, vegan diet.

You should tell your doctor what you plan to eat, especially if you are diabetic and on insulin. The doctor will be able to monitor your blood sugar levels and decrease medications when appropriate. When I told my doctor that I was going to eat a low-fat vegetarian diet, he laughed and told me that I could eat a vegetarian diet if I wanted to, but that it wouldn't affect my lupus.

When I first changed my diet, I really didn't know any of the science behind it. It seemed to make sense, and since nothing else had worked, I didn't see any harm in trying it. Now I know a little more about the underlying process of the immune system and will attempt to explain it in simple terms.

How the Immune System Works

Let's first look at how the body's immune system works. A healthy body has an immune system that is like a well-run army. One of the immune system's main functions is to constantly look for "foreign material" that doesn't belong in the body, which may harm the body or interfere with its many inner workings.

These foreign materials, called "antigens", can be many substances: viruses, bacteria, food, abnormal or dead cells, or environmental toxins.

When the immune system detects an antigen (foreign material) in the body, it produces an antibody which attaches itself to the antigen, forming an antigen-antibody complex (also called an immune complex).

The immune system then calls in other forces from its army to destroy these antigen-antibody complexes, and eliminate them from the body.

This is all part of a normally functioning immune system.

Now, let's look at what can go awry.

What goes wrong in the immune system and triggers Lupus?
Research shows that lupus occurs if:

- Immune system produces "too many" antigen-antibody complexes, which don't get destroyed, and become lodged in the body's tissues—causing inflammation and damage.
- Immune system produces autoantibodies (antibodies to self), which directly attack the body's tissues, causing inflammation and damage.
- Too many antigens and antigen-antibody complexes
- A problem occurs when too many antigens appear in the body, which results in the formation of too many antigen-antibody complexes.

These complexes circulate throughout the body, in the bloodstream. Sometimes the body can't clear the complexes because they are too large, too small or too plentiful.

If the body is unable to eliminate or clear these antigen-antibody complexes, they can become lodged in the body's tissues. They can be lodged almost anywhere, but most often in the joints, skin, kidneys, or other organs. Once lodged in the body's tissues, they cause irritation to the body, which results in inflammation and damage (similar to what happens when a wooden splinter gets stuck under your skin).

If antigen-antibody complexes become lodged in one of your joints, the joint becomes inflamed, and you'll have joint pain. If lodged in your kidney, the inflammation can cause abnormal kidney functioning. If the skin is inflamed, it can produce psoriasis. If the thyroid cells are inflamed, they are stimulated and cause excessive secretion of thyroid hormone, resulting in Grave's disease. When the inflammation is in the synovium (tissue lining the joint), it can create rheumatoid arthritis. In lupus, almost any system of the body can become inflamed, including the joints, muscles, skin, or organs like the kidneys, lungs, heart, brain or nervous system.

This is an abnormal immune response and happens when the immune system is unable to properly destroy and clear these antigen-antibody complexes.

Why Too Many Antigens and Antigen-Antibodies?

Why are there excess antigens in people with lupus? Some researchers and clinicians have discovered that a source of antigens can be from the foods we eat.

What? How could the body see food as a foreign invader? There are several reasons this could happen.

Increased intestinal permeability

The intestine is a barrier that keeps the contents of the foods you eat from the rest of the body. The intestine digests and absorbs nutrients from the foods you eat, and eliminates the rest. The digestive system is designed so that foods are contained inside the digestive tract from the mouth all the way to elimination through the anus. The actual food does not come in contact with the rest of your body.

In the digestive tract, food is broken down into small useable molecules, and these nutrients are absorbed by the body through the permeable membrane of the intestines.

In some people, this delicate membrane of the intestine is damaged and becomes permeable, allowing whole, undigested food molecules directly into the bloodstream.

Inflammation of the digestive tract can cause swelling, which pulls the cells of the digestive tract apart, creating more spaces between the cells. Damage to the gut lining can be from genetics, bacteria, infections, antibiotic use, inflammation of the intestine, overeating of refined carbohydrates, dietary fat and cholesterol.

Once the intestinal lining is damaged, undigested proteins can pass through it, allowing antigens (foreign material) into the body.

Ironically, anti-inflammatory drugs (NSAIDs) that many people with lupus take (such as Advil®, Motrin®, and Naprosyn®), have been shown to increase intestinal permeability.

Foreign proteins in the bloodstream

Through these intestinal openings, undigested proteins from foods and bacteria can leak into the bloodstream.

Normally, only small molecules are allowed through the intestinal wall into the rest of the body. Any large molecule that gets through is viewed by the body as an antigen, an "invader" that doesn't belong there.

There have been studies that show how easily undigested milk products can pass through the intestinal wall into the blood stream. This is why doctors advise against feeding cow's milk to babies. A baby's intestinal tract is very porous, which allows large protein molecules of human mother's milk through, ensuring adequate absorption of nutrients.

Excess antigen antibody complexes formed

These undigested proteins that get through the intestinal membrane are seen as invaders, and the immune system attacks, attaching an antibody to the antigen. This creates an antigen-antibody complex.

In lupus, and many other autoimmune disorders, the body accumulates more antigen-antibodies than it can destroy. They circulate in the blood stream and land in various tissues throughout the body, causing inflammation—much like a splinter stuck under the skin.

Arachidonic acid creates inflammation to joints and tissues

Animal fats contain large quantities of a fatty acid called arachidonic acid. The body converts this fatty acid into a chemical that inflames joints and tissues.

Immune response impaired by sludged up immune system

The normal clearing and removal of antigen-antibody complexes can also be impaired from too much fat and cholesterol in the bloodstream, which sludges up the blood and interferes with the effectiveness of the immune system. Studies have shown that both animal product fats and vegetable oils suppress the immune system.

Intestinal flora alteration

A study on the effects of a vegan diet and rheumatoid arthritis clearly showed that the bacterial composition of the feces of people on a vegan diet were significantly different from those on a carnivorous diet.

The people on the vegan diet showed improvement in their rheumatoid arthritis symptoms, where as those on the carnivorous diet did not improve.

These bacteria in the gut could be inflaming the intestinal tract, causing small openings. Both the bacteria itself as well as undigested proteins could be then escaping into to the body, creating antigens.

Why does the immune system create autoantibodies? (antibodies that directly attack your own tissues)

In addition to the excess of antigen-antibody complexes, another factor in autoimmune disease is the formation of autoantibodies. Autoantibodies are produced by the immune system and directly attack the body's normal cell tissue (not just foreign material), causing inflammation and damage.

Why would the body attack its own tissues?

It's not known why autoantibodies are formed, but it's likely that either the body's cells are altered and appear foreign, or that some part of the immune function is impaired.

Autoantibodies can attack almost anywhere—the DNA of the cell, the surface of the cell, white blood cells, or red blood cells. Some of the names of autoantibodies may be familiar to you if you've been tested for them: anti-DNA, anti-Sm, anti-RNP, and anti-La, to name just a few.

Molecular mimicry

Proteins that make up human tissue are very close in molecular structure to the proteins in animal tissue. It's thought that autoantibodies occur when the body attacks both the animal protein antigens and normal human tissue, which appears to be the same as the antigen.

As more antigen-antibody complexes become lodged in the tissues, the inflammation worsens. The body can become overwhelmed and start to produce autoantibodies.

Damage from lack of oxygen to the tissues

When blood is thick with fat and oil, the amount of oxygen that gets to the tissues is reduced, which causes tissue damage, and can cause the production of autoantibodies.

WHY DOES DIET MAKE A DIFFERENCE?

The foods that are most likely to pass through the intestinal wall and be seen as antigens by the body, are animal proteins—found in meat and dairy products. Some people also react to various plant proteins—common ones are wheat, corn and alfalfa.

Studies and clinical observations have shown that inflammation and autoimmune disease activity often significantly decrease when meat and dairy products are removed from a person's diet.

The amount of time it takes the existing inflammation to cool down differs with each person and with the severity of the disease activity.

Some people change their diet for a week or so and assume that foods are not a trigger when they don't feel an immediate improvement. Remember, you not only have to stop producing new antigens, but you must also allow time for the body to clear the antigen-antibody complexes that are already lodged in your tissues, and also time to calm the existing autoantibody activity.

It can sometimes be difficult to turn the autoantibody process around, but it is possible.

The first step is to stop eating foods that are creating antigens.

The second step is to give the body the time and energy it needs to clear antigen-antibody complexes that are already lodged in its tissues and stop the autoantibody process.

A low-fat, whole food, plant-based diet can:

- Decrease or eliminate foods that are creating antigens
- Decrease intestinal permeability (gut leakage)
- Provide foods that require less energy to digest, freeing up more energy for clearing existing immune complexes and calming auto-antibody activity
- Eliminate intake of animal fat and cholesterol
- Eliminate intake of animal proteins
- Increase intake of plant proteins
- Reduce intake of arachidonic acid
- Decrease excess sodium consumption (meat and dairy contain very high levels of sodium)
- Decrease over-consumption of Omega 6 fats—which cause inflammation
- Increase consumption of Omega 3 fats—which reduce inflammation
- Provide high level of antioxidants and phytochemicals
- Provide high volume of dietary fiber

Which then can:

- Decrease number of antigen-antibodies complexes formed
- Decrease inflammation and tissue damage
- Decrease joint pain
- Decrease strain on kidneys and spleen
- Lower blood pressure
- Lower cholesterol level
- Decrease risk of heart attack and stroke
- Normalize body weight
- Eliminate constipation

WHY ISN'T THE ROLE OF DIET BETTER KNOWN?

"Often diet and nutrition and lifestyle are perceived to be sort of passé or too simple, and yet they are very important topics. There is interesting science behind it, but because it's not regarded as so novel and new, it's often neglected in scientific funding."

— Dr. Walter Willett, MD, Harvard School of Public Health

"Imagine the publicity if someone announced that they have developed a new treatment that cured 40 percent of all people with cancer. The media would be jumping up and down. That kind of benefit can be achieved today just by following a vegetarian diet. Right there you have an answer and no one's listening."

—Oliver Alabaster, M.D., Oncologist, Director of the Institute for Disease Prevention, George Washington University

"You will observe with concern how long a truth may be known and exist, before it is generally received and practiced on."

— Benjamin Franklin

Sometimes things that are obvious to us now have not always been so obvious.

Not too many years ago, in the mid-1800s, two medical doctors discovered that doctors who washed their hands between surgeries significantly lowered the rate of death in their patients. Yet, these doctors were ridiculed and criticized for their discovery, and it took another twenty years before hand-washing became accepted as a necessary practice.

Up until the 1970s cigarette smoking was thought to be harmless—and some cigarette ads even highlighted doctors recommending their favorite brand. Smoking was sometimes prescribed for anxious patients. Today everyone knows how dangerous smoking is for your health.

There are doctors and scientists who feel that one day the consumption of meat and dairy will be seen as dangerous as cigarette smoking is seen today.

Why don't more people, including your doctor, know the major role that diet and lifestyle play in lupus and other autoimmune diseases? There are a multitude of reasons.

Medical Schools teach allopathic medicine.

The primary reason that your doctor is unaware of the dramatic effects of diet and lifestyle on autoimmune disease is that he or she has been taught *allopathic* medicine. *Allopathic* medicine focuses on *symptomatic* treatment. Physicians are taught how to treat illness by treating and suppressing the *symptoms*.

Symptomatic treatments suppress, stimulate, or relieve symptoms. A *symptomatic* treatment does not affect or remove the cause of the disease. There is definitely a place for symptomatic therapy, particularly in emergency, and life or limb threatening situations.

Doctors are not trained in diet or nutrition

Doctors generally receive fewer than three hours of nutritional training in medical school. They are not trained in nutrition or in health-promoting activities.

Most doctors eat the standard American diet themselves and don't have any idea how good a plant-based diet is for human health, and especially for someone with lupus.

Many doctors assume that their patients would not be willing to change their diets. Some doctors who have never tried a low-fat, vegan diet themselves have said that they thought that it would be too restrictive a diet to follow, and that their patients wouldn't be willing to do it either.

And in some cases they are right—there are some people who would rather take drugs than eat differently. But wouldn't you like to make that decision for yourself? One young girl who overcame lupus nephritis said, "I don't see how anyone could think that the effects of taking Prednisone and Cytoxan are easier than eating different foods. I'll do anything to stay off of those drugs."

Dietary studies are not popular with researchers

Numerous challenges are associated with clinical trials of dietary treatment. Many researchers do not want to undertake a dietary trial. They must recruit patients for the trial who are willing to make daily lifestyle changes, not just take a pill.

Compliance can be difficult to monitor unless the patients are in an in-patient environment. Also, it is difficult to conduct a double-blind study. In a double-blind study, neither the patient nor the examining doctor knows whether the person is receiving the drug or the placebo pill. In a dietary trial, obviously the patients know what food they are eating...or not eating.

Drug studies have financial backing

Drug trials are usually funded by a pharmaceutical company with a financial interest linked to the clinical trial, where as dietary studies are not.

Dr. Walter Willet, MD said in an interview with Frontline, "I think the government has under-funded research in diet and nutrition. In some ways we blame the abstract government for it, but in some sense it's also the scientific community that's partly to blame for it, because we often tend to fund the novel, exciting science, the new gene discoveries, the new mechanisms of drugs, for example."

Successful studies on diet and autoimmune disease don't get much attention.

There have been studies done on the effectiveness of diet and autoimmune disorders. Often diet and nutrition and lifestyle studies don't get much attention because they seem too simple, or are not exciting enough. Also, since there is not a product or drug to sell, there is not a marketing department to promote the results.

Broccoli and salad don't sound very exciting or sexy to the media. Some studies have shown exciting results with the effect of diet and autoimmune diseases, but they have been largely ignored. Plain and simple healthy living doesn't make headlines. If a drug could produce the results that a plant-based diet does— it would be in all the headlines.

Some fasting studies have concluded that the benefits are lost once eating resumes.

Some studies showed a return of symptoms after patients resumed eating. This happened in cases where they resumed eating dairy, meat or a high fat and oil content foods.

Several recent studies have shown that a vegan diet, with or without an initial period of fasting, has long-term significant benefit with many rheumatoid arthritis and lupus patients.

Some doctors have read of the positive effects of fasting on autoimmune disease, but don't know that supervised fasting is practical other than in a scientific study.

There are some doctors who have read the studies on the effects of diet and fasting on autoimmune disorders, but who do not realize that there are professional fasting centers that can medically supervise a water-only fast, with consistent, positive results.

Many doctors dismiss their patients' claims of diet-based improvements.

Some doctors don't know about the effects of diet because they don't listen to their patients who tell them that dietary changes made a difference. When I went back to my rheumatologist and told him of the specific steps I had taken, and the specific results I got—he wrote "spontaneous remission" in my chart. He had no interest in hearing about my experiences.

He worked and taught at the Medical College of Virginia—a university teaching hospital. Months earlier he had said, "You can eat anything that you want, but it doesn't have a thing to do with your lupus." It seemed that was his belief, and he was sticking to it, regardless of the results I had gotten. I never went back to him after that.

Very few people with lupus or rheumatoid arthritis have tried diet intervention.

The official word from the medical community is that diet has no effect on lupus or rheumatoid arthritis. Therefore very few people have researched it, or tried manipulating the foods they eat.

The few people who have experimented with diet, but without the right guidance, often fail to see good results. It takes a specific program of low-fat, vegan foods, like the program that is outlined in this book.

HAVE CLINICAL TRIALS AND STUDIES BEEN DONE?

Over the years, many clinical trials and studies have shown that dietary manipulation can significantly affect and improve the symptoms of rheumatoid arthritis and lupus.

Studies of clinical trials have been published on **Water-only fasts** (Fuhrman, 2002; Hafstrom, 1988; Kroker, 1984; Panush, 1986), **Vegetable and fruit juice-only fasts** (Lithell, 1983; Skoldstam,1979, 1991; Sundqvist, 1982), **Raw food diets** (Donaldson, 2001), **Elimination diets** (Darlington, 1986; Hicklin,1980; Kavanghi, 1995; van der Laar, 1992), **Lacto-vegetarian diets (includes dairy)** (Kjeldsen-Kragh, 1991; Skoldstam, 1979; Sundqvist et al., 1982), and **Vegan Diets (pure vegetarian)** (McDougall, 2002; Hafstrom, 2001, Beri, 1988; Darlington, 1991; Kjeldsen-Kragh, 1991; Nenonen, 1998; Parke,1981; Ratner,1985; Seignalet,1992).

For years, modified diets and fasting have been shown to be very effective at reducing the pain and inflammation of autoimmune disease. However, many of the studies reported a return of symptoms once the participants began eating an unrestricted diet (milk and dairy products or high fat foods, such as meats or processed vegetable oils).

Therefore up until recently, the prevailing opinion in the medical community was that fasting or modified diets were not effective in the long-term treatment of autoimmune disease.

However, more recent studies have confirmed that dietary modifications can have long- lasting benefits.

In 2001, Horst Muller, with the Baineology and Rehabilitation Science Research Institute in Germany, reviewed the previously reported scientific studies to see if long-term benefits could be maintained beyond an initial fast.

He found thirty-one published, controlled studies that investigated the effects of fasting on rheumatoid arthritis. Four were controlled studies that reported follow-up data for at least three months after the treatment.

Muller's study, published in the *Scandinavian Journal of Rheumatology*, states "Pooling of these studies showed a statistically and clinically beneficial long term effect." He concluded that available evidence suggested that fasting followed by vegetarian diet could be beneficial, and said there was an urgent need for additional studies.

In 2001, the journal *Rheumatology* published a study by Hafstrom. Sixty-six rheumatoid arthritis patients were enrolled in a one-year study. Thirty-eight were assigned to a gluten-free, vegan diet and twenty-eight to a non-vegan diet. The gluten free, vegan diet was used to eliminate the consumption of proteins from milk and grains that seemed to cause immune reaction in many people. Forty percent of people in vegan group improved, compared to just one person in the control group.

In 2001, Donaldson tested a mostly raw vegan diet in thirty patients with fibromyalgia. After several months on the diet, nineteen had significant improvement in range of motion, flexibility, and fatigue level. This study is mentioned because many people with lupus and rheumatoid arthritis also have a diagnosis of fibromyalgia. (*BMC Complement Altern Med, 2001*)

In October of 2001, the professional journal *Alternative Therapies* published case reports by Dr. Joel Fuhrman showing long-term remission of symptoms with water-only fasting and a low fat, vegan diet in six cases—including rheumatoid arthritis, systemic lupus and connective tissue disease.

After fasting from one to three weeks, the patients were free of symptoms, and their symptoms did not return when they resumed eating a low-fat, whole foods vegan diet. Remission was confirmed months and sometimes, years later.

In 2002 the *Journal of Alternative and Complementary Medicine* reported the findings of Dr. John McDougall. McDougall reviewed studies already published and from them hypothesized that a low fat, vegan diet would be an effective method of treatment for rheumatoid arthritis.

He wanted to measure the results of dietary changes, without fasting, as it can be too difficult or expensive for some people to undergo a medically supervised fast, or a clinically managed elimination diet.

The study evaluated twenty-four free-living individuals with rheumatoid arthritis. They met weekly for compliance and progress monitoring, as well as diet instruction. Pre-study and post-study evaluation was done by a rheumatologist who was unaware of the study design.

Twenty-two of the twenty-four patients completed the study. The study concluded "Patients with moderate to severe RA, who switch to a very low-fat, vegan diet can experience significant reductions in RA symptoms."

This study included wheat and cereals in the diet, and McDougall stated that the results could possibly have been even better if these foods were eliminated.

Additional studies in both The *Lancet* and *The Annals of Internal Medicine* showed good results when testing the effects of a low-fat diet on animals with lupus. Both researchers recommended that the results looked promising and that further dietary trials should be done on the effects of low-fat diets and low-animal protein diets for people with lupus.

The following compilation of studies is part of an article that Dr. John McDougall wrote entitled "Diet, the only Real Hope for Arthritis." An excerpt is reprinted here with permission from Dr. McDougall. The entire article can be viewed at www.drmcdougall.com/newsletter/may_june1.html

Diets Can Cure: The Research

Treatment of arthritis with diet had become fashionable in the 1920s and many studies over the last 20 years have shown that a healthy diet, one very different from the typical American diet, can be a very effective treatment of inflammatory arthritis for many people.

"One-third of the patients improved..."

In 1979, Skoldstam fasted 16 patients with rheumatoid arthritis for 7-10 days with a fruit and vegetable juice fast, followed by a lacto vegetarian diet for 9 weeks. One-third of the patients improved during the fast, but all deteriorated when the milk products were reintroduced (a lacto vegetarian diet) (*Scan J Rheumatol* 8:249, 1979).

"Food sensitivities reported..."

In 1980, Hicklin reported clinical improvement in 24 of 72 rheumatoid patients on an exclusion diet. Food sensitivities were reported to: grains in 14, milk in 4, nuts in 8, beef in 4, cheese in 7, eggs in 5, and one each to chicken, fish, potato, and liver (*Clin Allergy* 10:463, 1980).

"Wheat, corn and beef greatest offenders..."

In 1980, Stroud reported on 44 patients with rheumatoid arthritis treated with the elimination of food and chemical avoidance. They were then challenged with foods. Wheat, corn, and beef were the greatest offenders (*Clin Res* 28:791A, 1980).

"Recovered after stopping all dairy products..."

In 1981, Parke described a 38-year-old mother with 11-years of progressive erosive seronegative rheumatoid arthritis who recovered from her disease, attaining full mobility, by stopping all dairy products. She was then hospitalized and challenged with 3 pounds of cheese and seven pints of milk over 3 days. Within 24 hours there was a pronounced deterioration of the patient's arthritis (*BMJ* 282:2027, 1981).

"Fat-free diet produced complete remission..."

In 1981, Lucas found a fat-free diet produced complete remission in 6 patients with rheumatoid arthritis. Remission was lost within 24-72 hours of eating a high-fat meal, such as one containing chicken, cheese, safflower oil, beef, or coconut oil. The authors concluded, "...dietary fats in amounts normally eaten in the American diet cause the inflammatory joint changes seen in rheumatoid arthritis." (*Clin Res* 29:754, 1981).

"Fasting may ameliorate the disease activity..."

In 1982 Sundqvist studied the influence of fasting with 3 liters of fruit and vegetable juice daily and lacto vegetarian diet on intestinal permeability in 5 patients with rheumatoid arthritis. Intestinal permeability decreased after fasting, but increased again during a subsequent lacto vegetarian diet regime (dairy products and vegetables). Concomitantly it appeared that disease activity first decreased and then increased again. The authors conclude, "The results indicate that, unlike a lacto vegetarian diet, fasting may ameliorate the disease activity and reduce both the intestinal and the non-intestinal permeability in rheumatoid arthritis." (*Scand J Rheumatol* 11:33, 1982.)

"...during fasting, joint pains were less intense..."

In 1983, Lithell studied twenty patients with arthritis and various skin diseases on a metabolic ward during a 2-week period of modified fast on vegetarian broth and drinks, followed by a 3-week period of a vegan diet (no animal products). During fasting, joint pains were less intense in many subjects. In some types of skin diseases (pustulosis palmaris et plantaris and atopic eczema) an improvement could be demonstrated during the fast. During the vegan diet, both signs and symptoms returned in most patients, with the exception of some patients with psoriasis who experienced an improvement. The vegan diet was very high-fat (42% fat). (*Acta Derm Venereol* 63:397, 1983).

"The group improved significantly..."

In 1984 Kroker described 43 patients from three hospital centers who underwent a 1-week water fast, and overall the group improved significantly during the fast. In 31 patients evaluated, 25 had "fair" to "excellent" responses and 6 had "poor" responses. Those with more advanced arthritis had the poor responses. (*Clin Ecol* 2:137, 1984).

" ...7 out of 15 went into remission..."

In 1985, Ratner removed all dairy products from the diet of patients with seronegative rheumatoid arthritis, 7 out of 15 went into remission when switched to milk-free diets (*Isr J Med Sci* 21:532, 1985)

"No more morning stiffness..."

In 1986, Panush described a challenge of milk in a 52-year-old white woman with 11 years of active disease with exacerbations allegedly associated with meat, milk, and beans. After fasting (3 days) or taking Vivonex (2 days) there was no morning stiffness or swollen joints. Challenges with cow's milk (blinded in a capsule) brought all of her pain, swelling and stiffness back (*Arthritis Rheum* 29:220, 1986).

"41 out of 48 identified foods producing symptoms..."

In 1986, Darlington published a 6-week, placebo-controlled, single-blinded study on 48 patients. Forty-one patients identified foods producing symptoms. Cereal foods, such as corn and wheat gave symptoms in more than 50% of patients (*Lancet* 1:236, 1986).

"cow's milk produced significant joint lesions..."

In 1986, Hanglow performed a study of the comparison of the arthritis-inducing properties of cow's milk, egg protein and soymilk in experimental animals. The 12-week cow's milk feeding regimen produced the highest incidence of significant joint lesions. Egg protein was less arthritis-inducing than cow's milk, and soymilk caused no reaction. (*Int Arch Allergy Appl Immunol* 80:192, 1986).

"23 out of 41 improved..."

In 1987, Wojtulewski reported on 41 patients with rheumatoid arthritis treated with a 4-week elimination diet. Twenty-three improved. (*Food allergy and intolerance*. London: Bailliere Tindall 723, 1987).

"71% showed significant clinical improvement..."

In 1988, Beri put 14 patients with rheumatoid arthritis on a diet free from pulses, cereals, milk, and non-vegetarian protein foods. Ten (71%) showed significant clinical improvement. Only three patients (11%) adhered to the diet for a period of 10 months (*Ann Rheum* Dis 47:69, 1988.)

"morning stiffness and swollen joints decreased..."

In 1988, Hafstrom fasted 14 patients with water only for one week. During fasting the duration of morning stiffness, and number and size of swollen joints decreased in all 14 patients. No adverse effects of fasting were seen except transient weakness and lightheadedness. The authors consider fasting as one possible way to induce rapid improvement in rheumatoid arthritis (*Arthritis Rheum* 31:585, 1988).

"vegan diet....significant improvement..."

In 1991, Kjeldsen-Kragh put 27 patients on a modified fast with vegetable broths, followed by a vegan diet, and then a lacto-ovo vegetarian diet. Significant improvement occurred in objective and subjective parameters of their disease (*Lancet* 2:899, 1991) A two-year follow-up examination found all diet responders but only half of the diet non-responders still following the diet, further indicating that a group of patients with rheumatoid arthritis benefit from dietary manipulations and that the improvement can be sustained through a two-year period (*Clin Rheumatol* 13:475, 1994.) Patients dropping out with arthritic flares in the diet group left the study mainly when the lactovegetarian diet (dairy products) were introduced (*Lancet* 338:1209, 1991).

"one-third still well...without medication..."

In 1991 Darlington reported on 100 patients who had undergone dietary manipulation therapy in the past decade, one-third were still well and controlled on diet alone without any medication up to 7 ½ years after starting the diet treatment. They found most patients reacted to cereals and dairy products (*Lancet* 338:1209, 1991).

"almost all showed remarkable improvement..."

In 1991, Skoldstam fasted 15 patients for 7 to 10 days. Almost all of the patients showed remarkable improvement. Many patients felt the return of pain and stiffness on the day after returning to their "normal" eating and all benefit was lost after a week (*Rheum Dis Clin North Am* 17:363, 1991).

"favorable benefits appeared before the end of the third month..."

In 1992, Sheignalet reported on 46 adults with rheumatoid arthritis who eliminated dairy products and cereals. Thirty-six patients (78%) responded favorably with 17 clearly improved, and 19 in complete remission for one to five years. Eight of those 19 stopped all medications with no relapse. Favorable benefits appeared before the end of the third month in 32 of the patients (*Lancet* 339:68, 1992).

"intolerance for specific foodstuffs cited..."

In 1992, van de Laar showed benefits of a hypoallergenic, artificial diet in six rheumatoid patients. Placebo controlled rechallenges showed intolerance for specific foodstuffs in four patients. In two patients, biopsy of the joints showed specific (IgE) antibodies to certain foods (*Ann Rheum Dis* 51:303, 1992).

"vegetarian diet...kidney disease improved..."

In 1992, Shigemasa reported a 16-year-old girl with lupus who changed to a pure vegetarian diet (no animal foods) and stopped her steroids without her doctor's permission. After starting the diet her antibody titers (a reflection of disease activity) fell to normal and her kidney disease improved (*Lancet* 339:1177, 1992).

"reintroduction of food brought the symptoms back..."

In 1995, Kavanaghi showed an elemental diet (which is a hypoallergenic, protein-free, artificial diet consisting of essential amino acids, glucose, trace elements and vitamins) when given to 24 patients with rheumatoid arthritis improved their strength and arthritic symptoms. Reintroduction of food brought the old symptoms back (*Br J Rheumatol* 34:270, 1995).

"uncooked vegan diet decreased symptoms..."

In 1998, Nenonen tested the effects of an uncooked vegan diet, rich in lactobacilli, in rheumatoid patients randomized into diet and control groups. The intervention group experienced subjective relief of rheumatic symptoms during intervention. A return to an omnivorous diet aggravated symptoms. The results showed that an uncooked vegan diet, rich in lactobacilli, decreased subjective symptoms of rheumatoid arthritis (*Br J Rheumatol* 37:274, 1998).

Part Three: The Program

"I believe that diet plays a role in lupus control. A number of patients have allergies to certain foods, usually shown by an increase in joint pains. "

— Dr. Graham Hughes, M.D., Head of Lupus Research Center, St. Thomas Hospital, London, UK

"The science is clear. The results are unmistakable. Change your diet and dramatically reduce your risk of cancer, heart disease, diabetes and obesity."

—Dr. T. Colin Campbell, PhD, Professor Nutritional Biochemistry, Cornell University, Author of *"The China Study"*

THE PROGRAM

As you can see from the quotes at the start of this chapter, there is little disagreement among health practitioners that eating a healthy diet, getting enough sleep, engaging in moderate exercise and reducing stress are all beneficial in the management of the disease of lupus.

The controversy is in what constitutes a healthy diet, and **how much of an effect** diet, sleep, and exercise can have in the lupus (autoimmune) disease process.

Many people have found that diet, sleep and exercise can make a profound difference in how they feel.

Diet
- Eat a low-fat, whole-food, plant-based diet.
- Stop eating foods that can trigger an immune system response.

Sleep
- While trying to overcome lupus, sleep at least 8-10 hours a night.
- Deep levels of sleep are necessary for the body to release healing hormones.

Exercise
- Walk for ten to thirty minutes daily.
- The lymphatic system needs body movement to clear out antigen-antibody complexes and other wastes.
- Exercise also relieves body stress and helps you to sleep soundly.

Reduce Stress

- Quit pushing yourself through the day. Rest when you're tired. Use proven relaxation methods.
- Mental, physical, emotional, and chemical stress causes the body to produce excess adrenaline, which interferes with getting to the deep levels of sleep.

Period of Fasting

- Fasting is not always necessary, desired or appropriate, but has been shown to quickly reduce or eliminate pain and inflammation.

DIET—THE FOODS YOU EAT

Each person is at a different stage of disease and will improve at a different rate of speed. Some people are able to get significant benefits by eliminating just one offending food (such as dairy), while others need a water-only fast to stop the autoimmune process.

Regardless of the speed, the *Lupus Recovery Diet* consists of **Three Basic Steps**:

1. Stop eating foods that have been shown to create antigens in the human body.

2. Give your body the time and energy it needs to clear out lodged antigen-antibodies, stop auto-antibody activity, and reduce the existing inflammation.

3. Reintroduce foods slowly, one at a time, and determine which ones cause your immune system to over react.

These three steps can be achieved in a variety of ways. A seven-to-ten day supervised water-only fast has been shown to quickly accomplish the first two steps. Juice-only or vegetable broth-only fasts have also produced quick results with steps one and two.

For those who do not want to fast, or who are on medication and cannot fast, steps one and two can also quickly be accomplished with an "elimination diet". On an elimination diet you eat only fruit, green and yellow vegetables, brown rice and sweet potatoes. It is effective because the only foods eaten are those that very rarely create food antigens. An elimination diet usually shows results within three to twenty-one days.

Whether you fast or eat an elimination diet, once the inflammation is reduced and symptoms are significantly improved, the reintroduction of foods is a very important step.

A low-fat, vegan, whole foods diet has been shown to be effective at maintaining the benefits achieved from a fast on a long-term basis (a vegan diet is one that excludes any animal products, including all meat, fish, dairy and eggs). When reintroducing foods, it is important to eat one new food at a time, so that you can identify which foods are triggering the immune reaction.

For those people who want to start with a less restrictive program than fasting or an elimination diet, you can begin by eating a low-fat, vegan, whole foods diet (with or without wheat and corn).

Some people are able to accomplish all three steps by just following this simple and delicious diet. It will usually take longer for the symptoms to subside than when utilizing a fast or an elimination diet—but some people still see quick results.

Foods Most Likely to Cause Antigens:

The "4 Whites"—Dairy, Salt, Sugar, Flour

Many nutrition experts, as well as the people whose stories are in this book, have found that this simple rule helped them the most: Stop eating meat and the 4 whites. The 4 whites are dairy, salt, sugar, and white flour.

Dairy

If you want to implement the diet one step at a time, start by eliminating dairy. Dairy is one of the worst aggravators of lupus and similar arthritis symptoms. It contains excess cholesterol, fat and proteins. Many studies have shown a direct link between autoimmune disease and dairy.

Dairy includes all milk proteins (especially casein and lactalbumin) in diary products—including whey, buttermilk solids, skim milk solids, calcium caseinate, sodium caseinate, all milk-derived cheeses, yogurt, ice cream and milk chocolate.

I know that the first question you have is where are you going to get your calcium. The answer to that is covered in detail in the Nutrition chapter, but the quick answer is you can get calcium from the same place that cows get it, from leafy green plants. There is an abundance of calcium in all vegetables, beans, nuts, seeds and whole grains.

Most of the world's population lives without drinking milk and have *significantly less* calcium deficiency diseases—like osteoporosis and hip fractures—than the populations that do drink milk.

White flour

White flour has been stripped of its nutritional value. The fiber has been removed, along with most nutrients, and then it is supplemented with artificial nutrients. It is a high-calorie, low-nutrient food. It's food like this that gives carbohydrates a bad name.

Additionally, the proteins in wheat can be a real inflammatant for some people with autoimmune disease, so it's best to leave all forms of wheat out at first, and then, if desired, introduce whole-grain flour back in later.

Salt

Salt is good for preserving and embalming things. I don't think you want your body to be in that category. Most processed foods are packed in a lot of salt. That's one reason the products can sit on the shelf for months.

You'll easily meet your body's sodium requirement with the *naturally occurring* sodium that is in plant foods.

If you still want some salt on your food, sprinkle a little on top before you eat it—instead of adding salt while cooking. It takes about 30 days to lose the craving for salt.

Sugar

Refined sugar, white or brown, suppresses the immune system and causes a host of other problems. A can of soda contains ten teaspoons of refined sugar!

Meat

This means meat from all animals—beef, fowl, pork, fish, eggs. As you'll read in the nutrition chapter, even lean meat is still very high in fat, cholesterol and excess protein.

I already know your next question, where do you get your protein? That is also explained in detail in the Nutrition chapter, but the quick answer is that it is easy to get plenty of protein by eating whole plant foods. I'll bet you didn't know that 100 calories of broccoli has more protein than 100 calories of steak!

Actually, the opposite is a bigger problem—most people consume too much protein. Unlike fat, the body cannot store protein. If too much protein is eaten, the body must eliminate it. This strains the kidneys and the spleen.

Human infants are growing the fastest in their first two years of life. Mother's milk, which is designed to be the food for babies, is just 5% protein.

Oil

Most people aren't aware of the dangers of oil. Oil is not a whole food. It would take a lot of olives to make a tablespoon of olive oil. How many olives would you want to eat at one time? Foods in nature are designed with the correct ratios of nutrients for us to eat. When we process them before eating, our nutrient intake can get out of balance.

Studies have shown that processed oils, from both plant and animal sources, sludge up and slow down the blood and the immune system. Hydrogenated oils are absolute poison to your body. Even the Federal Government says that there is no safe level of hydrogenated oils. When you look closely at the ingredient list, you'll be surprised at how many processed foods have hydrogenated oils added.

When you wash dishes you can see the difference in animal fats, processed oils and naturally occurring plant fats. You have to scrub with soap to remove animal fat or processed oil from a plate. The same thing happens inside your body—those fats are hard to get rid of. However, you can just rinse off the naturally occurring oil from an avocado or fresh coconut.

Studies and personal experiences have shown that an exclusively plant-based diet (vegan), that is low-fat, wheat-free and gluten-free is a very effective way of reducing the inflammation and pain of lupus and rheumatoid arthritis.

There are people (you've read of some in this book) who can eat wheat and gluten foods and can still overcome their symptoms. However, many feel the best results come from eliminating these foods initially, and then adding them back once you have improved.

So, how can I stop the inflammation?

There are multiple ways to begin. Start where you feel most comfortable. Your first steps can range from just eliminating the 4 whites – to starting with a juice or all raw food diet.

Here are the **options** beginning with the most "aggressive" and usually most effective program – down to individual steps.

- Water-only fast
- Juice-only fast
- Raw fruits and vegetables
- Elimination diet
- Whole food, vegan diet with no added oil - *Excluding* wheat, gluten, corn or soy

- Whole food, vegan diet with no added oil - *Including* wheat, gluten, corn and/or soy
- Eliminate the 4 Whites (dairy, white flour, salt and sugar)
- Eliminate dairy products

I will now describe each to you in more detail:

Water-only fast

Studies and clinical experience have shown that fasting can be very effective at reducing pain and inflammation. When fasting is followed with a low-fat, vegan diet—benefits have been seen quickly and have been long lasting.

The quickest and most effective step is a medically supervised water fast. However, not everyone is a candidate for fasting. If you are currently taking medications, you would need to work with a doctor to taper off those medications before beginning a fast.

Some people have found that a short one-to-three day water-only fast is a great way to jump-start a new dietary program (can not do if you're taking medications). A longer water-only fast is a remarkable therapy—**but must only be done under medical supervision**. More details in the Fasting Chapter.

Juice-only and/or vegetable broth-only fast

Studies have shown that a seven to ten day liquid-only fast can significantly reduce inflammation. The juices can be either vegetable or fruit. They MUST be freshly made. This involves either juicing your own each day, or buying fresh juice daily.

The downside of juicing is that juicing removes much of the fiber from the fresh fruits and vegetables. There is a lot of preparation and clean-up time involved, as the juices must be freshly made. Bottled or frozen juices have been pasteurized (heated at high temperatures) and are not appropriate for a juice-only fast.

Vegetable broth is the liquid left over after simmering water and vegetables. There is a vegetable broth in the recipe section.

A few days of a juice, vegetable broth, or water-only fast can also be a great way to start a new diet—either an elimination diet or a vegan diet.

Eat all raw fruits and vegetables

Eating all fresh, uncooked fruits and vegetables is another option. Many have found that a few days or a few weeks of eating only fresh, uncooked foods can quickly bring about a reduction in inflammation.

Elimination Diet

The goal of an elimination diet is to stop eating the foods that are most likely to be producing new food antigens. The following foods comprise what is commonly called an "elimination diet." These foods are considered safe foods, in that they will not cause an antigen or allergic reaction in most people.

- Fresh uncooked vegetables, particularly leafy greens
- Fruit (fresh or cooked—except citrus fruit and citrus juices)
- Fresh fruit and vegetable juices (not canned or bottled or frozen)
- Cooked green, yellow and orange vegetables
- Sweet potatoes
- Brown rice
- No added oils or spices
- Beverage: water only

Once you begin eating other foods, it is important to add just one new food at a time, every couple of days. Then, if you react to a food, you will be able to identify which food caused the reaction.

Start a daily log, recording what you eat, drink and how you feel. It can be telling as to what foods aggravate you and which don't. Keep a list of safe foods and trigger foods.

Some people will feel significantly better after a two-week elimination diet. Other people will need to continue for a longer period of time.

Eliminate the 4 Whites

Quit eating dairy products, white flour, salt and processed – sugar, as discussed in detail on the previous few pages.

Eliminate just dairy products

As seen in several studies (and many people's experiences), just eliminating dairy (milk and cheese) can noticeably affect symptoms.

What do you eat on The Lupus Recovery Diet?

The Lupus Recovery Diet is a low-fat, whole food, vegan diet. What does that mean? Think fresh. Think salad. Think vegetables. Think fruit. Think whole foods.

A *low-fat, whole food, plant-based diet* is what many people have found to be the key in overcoming their lupus symptoms.

- Whole food, low fat, plant based (vegan) diet
- Free from all Dairy products
- Free from all meat, fish, fowl, eggs
- Free from added oil
- Free from white sugar, white flour and salt
- Corn free, wheat free soy free, and gluten free (though not necessary for all people)
- Free from processed foods

What are Whole Foods?

Whole foods are foods you would find when walking around in a garden or an orchard. Foods like fruits, vegetables, leafy greens, potatoes, squashes, beans, avocados, nuts, and seeds. (There are many delicious whole food suggestions in the recipe section; mango-orange smoothie, eggplant pate, sweet potato soup, chickpea curry, and grilled Portobello mushrooms to name a few.)

A whole food is one that is eaten just as it is found in nature. A baked potato is a whole food, whereas pasta is not a whole food. See the difference? Pasta is a processed food. It is made from wheat, which is processed into flour, which is processed into pasta. There are no pasta bushes growing in the garden. You have to process the grain into something other than how it was grown.

Keep in mind that 100% whole foods are very important during the initial recovery period. Once your inflammation has subsided, additional foods can be added back to see how they affect you (things like bread, pasta, and soy-based meat substitutes).

What do I eat?

Eat 60% to 80% of fresh and uncooked foods:
- Fresh salads
- Dark leafy greens
- Other vegetables
- Fresh, ripe fruits
- A few raw nuts and seeds

Eat 20 to 40%:
- Steamed, baked, broiled, or stir fried vegetables
- Steamed, baked, broiled starchy vegetables
- Beans, lentils, peas
- Brown rice or other whole grains (like quinoa, millet, oats, etc)

Does that sound too boring? Then, let's describe it differently:

Breakfast:
- Strawberry banana smoothie or
- Bowl of sliced bananas and strawberries

Lunch:
- Green leafy salad topped with mango and walnuts
- Black bean soup

Dinner:
- Guacamole with sliced zucchini as chips
- Green leafy salad
- Baked sweet potato with garlic roasted vegetables
- Orange avocado sauce

Sound more appetizing? These foods are also very simple to prepare. In the "Recipe" chapter there are many more simple whole food recipes.

Busy or too tired to cook? Whole foods can be fast foods!

Even those of you who are too exhausted and sick to expend any energy on preparing food can still easily eat this way. Lupus recovery foods can be very simple to prepare, and are healthy "fast foods".

Fruit only takes a second to wash off. You can eat fruit for any meal, along with some salad greens.

It only takes a minute to make a smoothie; you place bananas, frozen fruit, and a little water into a blender. Simpler still, just peel the bananas and eat them.

You can buy pre-washed lettuce and greens in a bag, or you can wash and prep enough lettuce at one time to last five days.

A potato or butternut squash can be rinsed, placed on a pan, and put in the oven to bake. You can even bake three or four at a time, and keep them in the fridge to warm up for meals. You can do the same with a large batch of brown rice.

A can of beans can quickly be heated up, or poured on a salad. Frozen vegetables steamed in a saucepan cook in only five to seven minutes. Many grocery stores or restaurants have ready-to-eat salad bars.

You—or a friend or family member—can make a couple of pots of soup on a Sunday, which then just need to be heated up during the week. You can also freeze most soups in small containers to eat later.

Raw nuts are available in bulk bins or bags, ready to eat.

Even Wendy's fast food restaurant sells baked potatoes with steamed broccoli and a salad.

Get the point? This literally can be a fast food diet.

Once you start feeling better, and you want to prepare more elaborate whole food meals, there are many delicious, simple vegetarian recipes.

I have created a video that shows how to select and prepare fresh, whole foods. All the dishes are very simple; once you see them you probably won't even need to follow a recipe. I've even won a few cooking contests with some of them. You can see clips of it at www.LupusRecoveryDiet.com/store.html

What if I don't feel better after eating a low fat, vegan diet for a few months?

Every person is unique. Each became sick through a different combination of genetic and environmental factors.

One person may have just been diagnosed with lupus, yet have raging inflammation in a vital organ. Another person may have suffered with lupus for years, but the inflammation is easy to reverse. Each situation is different.

Try not to become discouraged. If after following a low-fat, whole food vegan diet for a period of time, and you don't feel or see improvement, there are several options:

- Continue a low-fat vegan diet for a few more months, and stop eating all wheat, corn and products containing gluten (gluten is hidden in a lot of products).
- Eat an elimination diet—consisting of cooked or raw foods.
- Contact a doctor experienced in whole foods nutrition for personalized guidance.
- Undergo a period of medically supervised fasting; a vegetable broth/juice-only fast or a water-only fast.

There are some people who may be so sick that they cannot get relief from their symptoms. Their bodies have become so damaged from both the disease progression and toxic medications, that full recovery is not possible.

However, even in these serious cases, this low-fat, plant-based, whole food diet can still provide many benefits. People with lupus have a higher incidence of high cholesterol, heart attack and stroke.

The Lupus Recovery Diet is the type of diet that has been shown to reverse the buildup of cholesterol in the arteries, which can lead to heart attacks and strokes. Dr. Dean Ornish and his work at University of San Francisco Medical Center and Dr. Caldwell Essylton, MD at the Cleveland Clinic have both proven this in their remarkable work.

Remember in the individual stories you read, some people regained their health in 2 weeks, while some took two years.

Be patient with yourself on this journey, and read everything related that you can find.

OTHER IMPORTANT FACTORS: SLEEP, EXERCISE AND STRESS CONTROL

Diet is very important, but it's not the only factor. Also important are:

- Plenty of deep sleep- stages 3 and 4.
- Light exercise—helps the immune system circulate and pump wastes out of the body.
- Reduce stress in your life—stress drains needed energy and produces excess adrenaline which interferes with deep sleep.

Sleep

Sleep matters, and of course you probably have heard that before, but it's the type of sleep you get that can affect your healing. A deficiency of stage 3 and 4 sleep can cause major problems.

There are five stages of sleep, and we go through them in cycles. Each cycle lasts about ninety minutes. Stage one is light, with stage two being a little deeper. Stage 3 is where delta waves begin to be produced.

Delta waves are the slowest and most relaxed brain waves. Stage 4 is the deepest and most relaxed stage of sleep. Each night, we normally spend from twenty to forty-five minutes in stage four sleep. REM (rapid eye movement) stage is next, where most dreaming occurs.

Delta wave sleep, found in sleep stages 3 and 4, is when the body releases the most important healing hormones, like testosterone and growth hormone. If you sleep long enough and deep enough at night, these hormones are produced.

In the 1970's, a psychiatrist did sleep studies on people with fibromyalgia. He measured their brain waves during sleep with the use of an EEG machine. He found that those with fibromyalgia spent very little time in stage 4 sleep.

Using this information, he found that in only a few days, he could create fibrositis (now called fibromyalgia) in healthy subjects, by gently stimulating them out of stage 4 sleep. When he stopped interfering with their sleep, they recovered, but only after they had slept longer than normal time in stage 4 sleep.

When you push yourself hard, either emotionally, physically, mentally or chemically, your body produces adrenaline. Excess adrenaline interferes with your sleep, and also interferes with the release of healing hormones.

The more tired you are, and the more you push, the more adrenaline you produce. This affects your sleep, particularly getting to those deep stages. You then wake up tired, and you have to push even harder to get through the day, which causes the body to produce even more adrenalin.

See how this can quickly become a cycle? So to stop the cycle, quit pushing and forcing yourself to function when you are too tired. Catch up on your sleep. Get more of that healing, restful, deep sleep. Get to sleep by 10 pm (at the latest) and sleep eight to ten hours each night.

Caffeine or alcohol can be real detriments to your healing. They are artificial chemical stimulants that interfere with deep levels of sleep.

The nervous system controls every cell and function in your body. When your energy is low and the nervous system is tired, nothing functions normally.

If your body is exhausted, it doesn't have the energy to heal and clean. Give yourself permission to sleep, and go to bed as early as you can.

Exercise

Everyone knows the general health benefits of exercise and that it strengthens your heart, your lungs, your muscles, and your bones.

You may not be aware of the important role that exercise plays in the workings of the immune system.

Unlike blood, which is pumped through your veins by the heart, the immune system and lymphatic fluid have no pump. The immune system is connected through a series of tiny capillaries, which carry a whitish lymphatic fluid. The movement and activity of your muscles are what circulate this fluid. Moderate exercise helps to circulate this lymph fluid and keep the immune system working properly.

Movement and exercise are so important to the proper working of your body's immune system. They help the lymphatic system pump out built up toxins and waste. They help your digestive and elimination systems work effectively.

It is important to do some type of physical movement, even if it is just for a few minutes a day. If inactive for a long time, the lymph does not flow well enough to flush away normal waste products. Poor circulation to and from the tissues is a primary contributor to disease.

Exercise also helps the body overcome stress, which in turn can help the immune system's functioning. It can also lead to better sleep.

Many of the people in this book feel that walking or some other form of exercise significantly helped in their recovery. Walking seems to be one of the simplest and most effective exercises. Swimming or light aerobics are also great.

But if you don't like to walk or it's not convenient for you to do—a mini trampoline is a fun thing to lightly bounce or jog on. You can even exercise on it while watching TV. I bounce on a rebounder every day, even if just for a few minutes.

Stress Reduction

Mental, physical, emotional, and chemical stress causes your body to produce excess adrenaline.

Stress is known to decrease immune function. Many of the people in the recovery stories shared that they were under a great deal of stress when they became ill or when their illness worsened.

I know that when I first became sick, I had been under a great deal of stress, some positive and some negative, but still stressful on the nervous system.

Since my recovery, I have been through some very stressful periods, but the stress alone has not caused the lupus to flare or return. It has been my experience that stress was the final blow on top of my already weakened body, but that stress alone does not cause the symptoms to return.

There is some stress that you do have control over, the stress that you've designed into your daily life. Start by evaluating your job. I used to commute three hours a day to and from work. That was such a waste of time and energy. I had to wake up very early in the morning, and got to sleep much too late at night, resulting in sleep deficiency.

Is your job a major stressor? Is there anything you can do to change that? Can you work a job that has fewer hours? Travel less? Can you move closer to where you work or work closer to home?

People have found that listening to relaxing music, stretching, exercise, biofeedback training, guided imagery, meditation or yoga can help reduce stress. It's also helpful to listen to a relaxation tape just before going to bed or at breaks during the day.

It would also help to take a true vacation...one without calls into work, crowds of people, and lots of noisy diversions.

Once you start feeling what true peace and relaxation is, you'll want more of it.

How Do I Stick with It?

Here are some suggestions:

Belief Level

Belief level is the key. You hear so much conflicting information that it's hard to know what to do. Would you really care about changing the foods you eat if you KNEW it would get rid of your lupus?

That is probably the biggest advantage to a water-only fast. Many people get immediate results, which raises your belief and commitment levels.

Restrictive Foods
- Look at it as a temporary situation—a trial run.
- Don't think of it as restrictive—but a "special" diet.
- You will learn to like eating this way—your taste buds adapt, and the food tastes great.

At Home
- Don't bring junk food in the house.
- Eat slowly, chew food thoroughly—this will increase the digestibility.
- Eat in a relaxed atmosphere—noise and stress can reduce digestive function.
- Eat the less concentrated foods, like salad, first—to be sure that you eat them.
- Keep meals simple.
- Eat for the right reason—hunger.
- Center entertainment around activities other than food.
- Exercise more, especially outdoors.
- Cultivate friendships with people who live healthfully. Supportive friends really help.

- Plan menus. It saves shopping and cooking time, and ensures that you always have something good and healthy to eat.
- Family meals - make it a family affair if possible.
- Involve the whole family. If family members have excess weight they'd like to lose, high blood pressure, high cholesterol, cancer, arthritis, constipation, eating the foods that are good for you will help them too.
- You can also make the same food for the whole family, and just add extra ingredients to theirs.
- Have someone else in the family take over the cooking for a few weeks or a month.

Eating Out
- Choose ethnic restaurants such as Chinese, Thai, Indian, or Japanese as they usually have many vegetable choices.
- Choose a place to eat that has a salad bar.
- Most restaurants can serve steamed vegetables and baked potatoes.
- Keep your order as simple as possible.
- Remember you are not seeking the approval of the waiter, the chef or your companions.
- Use lemon as a dressing.
- Bring your own delicious dressing in a tightly sealed container.

Social Situations
- Don't go out hungry—eat something first—so you aren't too hungry when you arrive. This can help you make good decisions on what to eat.
- Offer to bring a dish or the salad.
- Tell people your doctor has put you on a "special" diet.
- Tell people that you are allergic to certain foods.
- Don't draw attention to yourself.

- Change the subject about your food—get the person talking about themselves.

Other tips

Don't eat after 6 pm or 7 pm. Your food will digest better, you'll sleep better. You'll wake up in the morning feeling light. This will lighten the work on your digestive system.

In the morning:
- Drink 2 glasses of water (a little added lemon tastes great) when you first get up.
- Walk outside for ten to thirty minutes, the fresh air and exercise are so stimulating.
- Eat fruit for breakfast.

Journal pages

Keep a daily log of the food, exercise, and sleep. Note how you feel before and after eating. This can be very revealing.

Part Four: Is This a Balanced Diet?

"It is the position of the American Dietetic Association and Dieticians of Canada that appropriately planned vegetarian diets are healthful, nutritionally adequate, and provide health benefits in the prevention and treatment of certain diseases."
— American Dietetic Association

"It's easy to meet your nutrient requirements on a vegan diet. Protein, calcium, and iron are widely distributed in vegetables, whole grains, and legumes so building your diet from these foods makes getting enough of these nutrients no problem at all.

Entirely plant-based diets are naturally richer in fiber, folate, vitamin C and other important disease-fighting nutrients and phytochemicals than omnivorous ones. Choosing to set aside meats, eggs, and dairy products, not only often provides relief from chronic pain, it makes eating healthfully much simpler."
— Amy Joy Lanou, Ph.D. Nutrition Director, Physicians Committee for Responsible Medicine

Is a Plant Based Diet a Balanced Diet?

Some of you may be concerned about how healthy an all plant (vegan) diet is. Where do you get your protein? Where do you get your calcium? The answers may surprise you. As you see by the quotes above, there are many reputable sources that whole-heartedly recommend a plant-based diet.

There are big businesses trying to convince us that their products are what we need to meet our nutritional needs. There is so much conflicting and inaccurate information that it is hard to know what to believe.

My purpose in this chapter is to provide general information that will address the most frequently asked questions about the nutrition in a plant-based diet. I don't want you, your doctor or your family to immediately dismiss the Lupus Recovery Diet, assuming that a plant-based diet is not a healthy one. For more detailed nutritional information, see the nutrition section in the Resources chapter.

Most doctors who have actually studied plant-based nutrition end up eating this way themselves, and are proponents of its value.

Though food is part of many social and religious practices, basically we eat to survive. There are some requirements of life that we can only get through food. We need calories for fuel, protein, essential fatty acids, vitamins, minerals, fiber and water.

Where Do You Get Your Protein?

"Which do you think has more protein, a hamburger or broccoli? Per 100 calories, broccoli has 12.5 grams of protein, and hamburger has 9.5 grams."

—Health Science Magazine

"The beef industry has contributed to more deaths than all the wars of the century, all natural disasters, and all automobile accidents combined. If beef is your idea of 'real food for real people,' you'd better live real close to a real hospital."

—Dr. Neal Barnard, President, Physicians Committee for Responsible Medicine

Where do you get your protein? This is the first question that someone usually asks regarding a plant-based or vegetarian diet. The meat and dairy industry have done an excellent job at selling the need for their products. It is easy for them to market this message, as they receive millions in government subsidies every year.

Think about this...where do the strongest mammals on earth get their protein? The elephant, water buffalo, or horse? They get their protein from leafy green plants. Protein is abundantly available in plant foods.

Human mother's milk contains just 5% of its calories from protein. This is a baby's food when it doubles in size in just four to six months.

The U.S. government's recommended daily allowance (RDA) of protein is 0.8 grams per kilogram of lean (ideal) body weight. That translates to about 44 grams for an average adult female and 56 grams for an average adult male. The RDAs were based on studies that demonstrated the actual human need for protein to be much lower—only about 0.3 grams (15 to 20 grams daily).

The RDA was set higher than studies actually showed, because they wanted to insure that everyone, no matter what their physical condition, would get enough protein on this recommendation. This is a recommended amount—not a minimum requirement.

Most people eat too much protein. The typical American eats more than 100 grams of protein daily. Your body does not store excess protein, so it must be excreted through urine and feces. This causes extra work on the body, particularly the kidneys.

As many lupus patients develop kidney involvement, excess protein is an important issue. There are many more health problems from excess protein, than from a lack of it.

Take a look at the amount of protein in various foods:

Food	Protein (as percent of calories)
banana	5%
watermelon	8%
brown rice	9%
baked potato	13%
rolled oats	13%
lentils	36%
broccoli	45%
spinach	51%

It is almost impossible to eat a low-fat, whole food, plant-based diet, and not get enough protein, as long as you eat enough calories for your needs. Protein deficiencies are seen in people who are actually starving, because they are not getting enough food to eat.

Your body does not utilize protein in the same form that you eat it. Protein doesn't stick to your body just as you eat it (though excess fat does work this way). The body breaks food down into its separate amino acids, and then builds its own proteins.

Plants contain all of the essential amino acids that your body needs. Some plant foods have more of one type than another. You are able to get all of your protein requirements from plants. If you ate nothing but potatoes or brown rice, and ate enough of them to meet your caloric needs, you'd get enough protein.

There is a myth that proteins found in plant foods are "incomplete" proteins, and that two or more plant foods must be eaten together to be "complete" proteins. This has been scientifically proven to be inaccurate, but many uninformed people still repeat this old myth.

Where Do You Get Your Calcium?

"There's no reason to drink cow's milk at any time in your life. It was designed for calves, not humans, and we should all stop drinking it today."

—Dr. Frank A. Oski, former Director of Pediatrics, Johns Hopkins University

Calcium is a very important nutrient, but dairy products are not the best source of calcium, as they also contain high levels of fat, sodium, protein and cholesterol.

There is abundant calcium in plant foods, particularly in green vegetables. All unprocessed natural foods are calcium rich; even a whole orange has about 60 mg of calcium. Not only is the percentage of calcium high in plant foods, but also a higher percentage of the calcium can be absorbed and used by the body as compared to the calcium in dairy.

Calcium deficiencies are usually caused by calcium excretion, not from low intake of calcium. Research has shown that the acid in animal proteins, salt, refined sugar, and alcohol all cause your body to leech calcium from your bones in order to offset the acid and maintain the necessary alkalinity of the body.

Your bones can't retain calcium, no matter how much you consume, if you are consuming too much protein, salt, sugar or alcohol. Therefore, eating dairy can actually cause your bones to lose calcium. Makes you look at that milk mustache a little differently, eh?

Who drinks milk? Lots of species do. Dogs do. Rats do. Deer do. Cows do. Humans do. Milk is produced by the mother for her own babies. Dogs don't drink deer milk. There is no mammal on earth that drinks the milk of another species, except (some) humans. Milk is tailor made for its own kind. Cow's milk has the nutrients to turn a one hundred-pound calf into a four to six hundred-pound cow in less than a year. There is no other mammal on earth that continues to drink milk after it has been weaned.

Most of the world's human population doesn't drink milk, other than their own mother's milk as infants. The countries that consume the most dairy products have the highest rates of hip fractures and osteoporosis (with the USA near the top of the list). If drinking milk and eating cheese were a good source of calcium, the United States would not have such high rates of osteoporosis and hip fractures.

Food	Calcium (milligrams)
1 apple	10
1 cup romaine lettuce	20
1 baked potato	20
1 tablespoon almond butter	43
1 orange	56
1 cup chickpeas	78
1 cup butternut squash	84
1 cup kale	94
1 cup black beans	100
1 cup collards	148
1 cup broccoli	178

What about other essential nutrients?

Essential Fatty Acids

Most people eat too much fat in general, and specifically too much of the wrong type of fats. But, scientific research shows that too little of healthful fats can also be a problem. The fats that you need to consume are called essential fatty acids (EFAs). In the right amount and balance, these are good fats. The two essential fatty acids are alpha-linolenic acid, an Omega 3 fatty acid and linoleic acid, an Omega 6 fatty acid.

They are called essential fatty acids because they are, under most circumstances, the only two fatty acids that your body cannot produce for itself. Therefore, you must eat foods that contain them. Generally speaking, all of the other fats that your body needs can be made from these two EFAs.

Omega 6 fats are less susceptible to oxidative damage than Omega 3 fats, and therefore give foods a longer shelf life. Most people on the SAD (standard American diet) eat too many processed foods that contain lots of Omega 6 fats and not enough foods rich in Omega 3 fats. Inflammation and disease can result from this imbalance. You can limit Omega 6 fats by cutting out animal products; hydrogenated vegetable oils (as found in most margarines); as well as corn, cottonseed, safflower, sesame and soy oils typically found in processed foods.

You can get ample Omega 3 and Omega 6 fats (in the right balance) from a varied, whole foods, plant based diet that includes ground flax seeds, walnuts, leafy greens, nuts and seeds.

Most fruits and vegetables also contain both EFAs, but in smaller quantities. However, when a large percentage of your diet comes from fruits and vegetables, you can obtain adequate amounts of EFAs from them as well.

The fats are in these whole foods; therefore it is not necessary to extract them as oils. However, extracted oils (such as flax oil or fish oil) are sometimes used beneficially to correct fatty acid imbalances and help reduce inflammation. For example, flax oil and fish oil contain high levels of anti-inflammatory Omega 3 fats. Once a healthy diet is adopted with the correct amount and ratio of these two essential fats—you would usually no longer need these oils.

Vitamin B_{12}

B12 it is an essential nutrient, and humans need just small amounts of it.

All animal flesh contains B12, including our own. Therefore when you eat animal products, you eat B12. Vitamin B12 is found in bacteria in the soil.

Animals eat B12 when they pull greens from the earth that are covered in soil. Years ago, when humans ate foods right from the soil, and drank water from the streams, it was easy to eat bacteria and get enough B_{12}. Now that water is chlorinated and foods are thoroughly washed and processed, a person who is not eating bacteria from meat may need an outside source of B12.

There are people who are deficient in B12, even though they eat meat. This occurs because of problems with absorption and digestion. It is very easy to take a weekly B_{12} supplement, to insure that you are getting your requirement of this essential nutrient.

Vitamin D

Vitamin D is often called the sunshine vitamin. It is not found naturally in any food product—plant or animal. It is a vitamin that is manufactured by your own body in response to exposure to sunshine. However, some processed foods are supplemented with Vitamin D. Milk is an example of a food that is promoted for its vitamin D, yet it is artificially added to milk.

If you must avoid the sun because of a lupus sensitivity to sun, you can eat plant-based foods that are fortified with vitamin D or take a vitamin D supplement.

Folic acid (folate)

Folacin (folic acid) is an important part of red blood cell development, so as you might expect, a deficiency of it leads to anemia. The word folacin comes from foliage, which is the leaf system of plants, because the richest sources of the vitamin are green leafy vegetables.

The RDA of folacin is 400 micrograms. One hundred calories of raw spinach contains 908 micrograms, romaine lettuce 844, cooked spinach 639, raw broccoli and cabbage 250 micrograms, and cooked cabbage 97. To put that in context, uncooked vegetables have about one hundred calories per pound, and cooked vegetables are approximately three hundred calories per pound. It is easy to eat a half-pound of leafy green salad daily.

What About the Food Pyramid?

The four food groups were introduced in 1956 by the U.S. Department of Agriculture. Their mission was to promote the sale and consumption of meat and dairy products.

They distributed posters for school children teaching four food groups—meat, dairy, grains with fruit and vegetables sharing a group. This was taught to children for years, who then grew up teaching their children the same thing. Since two of the four groups contained livestock products, meals have become loaded with fat and cholesterol.

The meat and dairy lobbyists are so powerful, that it took a long time to change the format from its original 4 food groups to the revised pyramid today. The government subsidizes the meat and dairy industries, just as it did the tobacco industry (the tobacco subsidies are just now ending).

Will I Be a Skinny-Looking Weakling?

In case you still picture someone who eats a vegetarian diet as a skinny weakling, here are just a few well-known, athletic and robust vegetarians.

A partial list of famous vegetarian athletes:

- Ridgely Abele, eight national karate championships
- Peter Burwash, tennis champion, Davis cup winner
- Andres Cahling, Swedish body builder, Olympic gold in ski jump
- Chris Campbell, Olympic wrestler
- Nickey Cole, first woman to walk to North Pole
- Ruth Heidrich, six-time Ironwoman
- Keith Holmes, world-champion middle weight boxer
- Desmond Howard, professional football star, Heisman trophy winner
- Carl Lewis, Olympic runner and gold medallist
- Bill Manetti, power lifting champion
- Martina Navratilova, champion tennis player (still competing in major tournaments at age forty-seven)
- Bill Pearl, weight lifter and four time Mr. Universe
- Dave Scott, six-time winner of the Ironman triathlon
- Art Still, Buffalo Bills and Kansas City MVP defensive end, KS Hall of Fame
- Hank Aaron, baseball player
- Billie Jean King, champion tennis player
- And numerous others...

Part Five: Fasting

"Significant improvement may be obtained in rheumatoid arthritis patients by fasting followed by a vegetarian diet for one year."

—J. Kjeldsen-Kragh, Institute of Immunology and Rheumatology, National Hospital, Oslo, Norway

"A wonderful thing about fasting is that it puts an interval between the behavior you are accustomed to and the behavior that you aspire to."

—Dr. Ralph Cinque, DC

WHAT IS FASTING?

This chapter describes something that some people may find difficult to believe. I had the same thoughts when I first read about water-only fasting.

Before we talk about fasting, let's define it. Water-only fasting is the complete abstinence from all substances except pure water in an environment of complete rest. Fasting can last several days or even several weeks.

Water-only fasting should never be tried on your own, and should only be done with medical supervision. Many people are not good candidates for water-only fasting, and would first need months of medical care and dietary modifications before a fast could be considered. People taking medications are not able to fast, and need to work with a doctor to slowly taper off of medications before a fast could even be considered. Doctors who are experienced with water-only fasting are listed at the end of this section.

Now that we all understand that water-only fasting is done only with medical supervision, let's talk more about it.

It may sound absurd that abstaining from food could help to improve your health. It probably seems counterintuitive to survival.

Fasting is not new

Many people have fasted, for religious, political and health reasons. In the Bible, David, Jesus, and Elijah fasted for up to forty days. Socrates, Plato, Pythagoras, and Hippocrates (often called the Father of Western Medicine) all recommended fasting at times.

In 1877, Dr. Henry Tanner, a middle aged physician, decided that he wanted to die. He had suffered for years with rheumatism and allergies, and spent his days and nights in constant pain. He and his fellow physicians had determined that his case was hopeless.

Dr. Tanner had been taught in medical school that the body could only live for ten days without food. Since he didn't believe in suicide, he decided he would just go to bed, stop eating, and quietly die. He later stated "Life to me under those circumstances was not living...and I had made up my mind to rest from physical suffering in the arms of death."

By the fifth day of his fast, he began to sleep more peacefully. By the eleventh day, he felt "as well as in my youthful days." He was very confused about what was happening, and called Dr. Moyer, a fellow physician. Once Dr. Moyer had examined him, he said Tanner should be at death's door, but that instead he had never seen him look better. Tanner continued to fast, under Moyer's supervision, for another thirty-one days, for a total of forty-two days.

When Dr. Tanner's fellow physicians heard his story, he was highly criticized and accused of fraud. However, Dr. Tanner had the last laugh, as he lived to age ninety without rheumatism, allergies or chronic pain.

After I fast, can I eat anything I want to?

Fasting is part of a healthy lifestyle; it is not in place of one. It does not do any good to fast, and then return to the same diet and lifestyle you had previously. There is no sense in undergoing a fast if your intention is to go back to your previous way of eating.

Complete rest during a fast is important. Activity can double caloric usage and reduce the effectiveness of the fast. Rest is critical to ensure that a fast is both a safe and an effective experience.

In the wild, animals rest and fast when they are acutely ill. So do we. If you think about it, often you lose your appetite when you are sick with a cold or a headache.

When we're not acutely ill, the idea of fasting seems absurd. It goes against our programming, which encourages us to get enough food in order to survive. In our society we're urged to eat so that we can "get better". Even if you're lying on a hospital bed, food is brought to your lips.

Fasting removes all outside interference so that the body can heal using its built-in healing mechanisms.

Benefits of Fasting

There are many reasons that fasting can be beneficial to people suffering with autoimmune disease. Fasting can:
- Stop intake of food that may be causing dietary antigens
- Reduce inflammation
- Rapidly eliminate pain
- Clear out lodged immune complexes
- Stop autoantibody production
- Reduce gut leakage
- Ensure you get needed rest, relaxation, and sleep
- Ease the transition to making needed lifestyle changes
- Help taste buds reset so that simple, healthy foods taste good
- Allow you to introduce foods, one at a time, and see how the body reacts to them
- Motivate you to eat a healthy diet, as you see immediate results

Medically Supervised Fast

In order for a fast to be safe and effective, you should only do one under the care of a doctor who is experienced and trained in fasting supervision. Some people actually feel worse before they feel better. This is known as a "healing crisis." When medically supervised, the doctor will know the difference between a healing crisis and a problem that requires termination of the fast.

Medical supervision also provides a supportive environment. This ensures that you get the necessary rest and relaxation, and helps you to stay motivated to continue.

Hunger during a fast

Most people assume that they would be hungry, even ravenous, during the entire fast. Surprisingly, after a couple of days, the hunger sensation goes away. Since the body burns fat as its fuel when fasting, the appetite center becomes temporarily desensitized to glucose. This allows most people to fast comfortably for a couple of weeks or longer.

Fasting, not starving

There is an important difference between fasting and starving. Fasting is a period of abstinence of food during which the body's nutrient reserves are adequate to meet the body's nutritional needs.

Starvation occurs when the body's nutrient needs are not being met. There have been medically supervised fasts of over one-hundred days—with people who were overweight and had plenty of nutrient reserves.

Activity during fasting

There should be little, if any, activity during a fast. It is a time for both physical and mental rest. If you try to go about your daily activities, the body would become exhausted and start using the wrong fuels, such as burning muscle instead of fat reserves. This is a time to sleep, rest with your eyes closed, and catch up with reading, writing or watching movies.

Rest and Relaxation

The most important thing to remember about fasting is that it is just a time of rest and relaxation for your body—so that it can heal itself. You are not forcing the body to do anything, just giving it the space to use its own built-in healing mechanisms.

More on Fasting

I highly recommend that you read Dr. Fuhrman's book, *Fasting and Eating for Health*, and read Dr. Goldhamer's fasting articles at www.healthpromoting.com/Articles.

There are several fasting centers where you can undergo a supervised fast. I went to TrueNorth Health Education Center in Rohnert Park, CA. They have conducted more than five thousand fasts since 1984, and have a staff of competent and experienced doctors. There can be up to twenty people fasting at one time, so there is plenty of motivation and encouragement.

Even though the staff joke about it being a prison, and you pay them to lock you up and not feed you, you are in control—and can stop a fast anytime that you want to.

They provide health education, with daily videos and lectures. You receive an excellent education while there, so that you know what to do when you return home.

Personally, I struggled with staying on a "clean" diet until after I fasted. The fast had such dramatic results for me in such a short period of time, that I was convinced beyond all doubt that food was a major culprit in my disease.

After fasting, I quickly became a believer in my body's ability to heal. I was so motivated to continue feeling great—that I would have eaten sawdust if that's what was necessary. Luckily, I found that whole natural foods tasted great, and that I didn't need to resort to sawdust.

DETAILS OF JILL'S FASTING EXPERIENCE

Each day during my long work commute, I listened to recordings from natural health conferences. After listening to these tapes for hours, I felt that I knew the speakers personally. Eventually I called Dr. Goldhamer and talked about my condition and what the options were. He had encouraging things to say about what he had seen with lupus and water-only fasting.

It still took me a few months to decide to fast. It was a big commitment to take three weeks off from work, and travel from Virginia to California. I didn't have anyone that I could talk with about fasting. My friends thought it sounded crazy.

Once I decided to fast I didn't tell too many people. I told work that I was going to a retreat center for lupus treatments. They didn't question it, as it was obvious by the way I limped around the office that I was sick and needed help.

The TrueNorth Health fasting center is in Rohnert Park, California—about one and a half-hours north of San Francisco. The flight from Virginia and subsequent bus connections took an entire day. By the time I arrived at TrueNorth, I couldn't even open the cab door. I had to be helped to my room. It felt so good to lie down and know that I didn't have to do anything—not work, not talk—not even eat!

On their recommendation, I had eaten all raw food for three days prior to arriving at the center. This ensures a high level of fiber and helps to clear your bowels before the fast begins. If you don't eat a few days of just fruit and salad before you arrive, they will feed you those foods for a couple of days before you start the fast. The "cleaner" you eat before the fast, the easier the fast goes. Those people who stop off at McDonald's before the fast regret it later.

I began to fast in June of 1995. The lab work on that first morning showed that my sed rate was 98. This means that there was a lot of inflammation in my body. Understandably, I was in a lot of pain and utterly exhausted. If I hadn't started the fast then, I would have had to begin steroidal treatment.

Each day a doctor would make morning and evening rounds. They checked my pulse, blood pressure, temperature, pupils, and general alertness. They also did urine and blood tests weekly. There is someone on site twenty-four hours in case you need assistance.

By the seventh day of the water fast—I had no joint pain. Let me repeat that. No joint pain—after three years of living with it every day. I was amazed and overjoyed! There are not words to describe how happy I was.

I continued with the fast for a total of fourteen days, as originally planned. By the end of the fast, my face was a beautiful, cool white—instead of that blazing red that it been for the previous few years. I lost about fourteen pounds of excess weight, and looked and felt great.

I did have some other uncomfortable things happen while fasting. Every day, the joint pain was diminishing, but there were other "healing crisis" events. Your body dumps out built up waste and toxins from years of accumulation. They can be expelled from any orifice of your body. Yes, it can be pretty ugly and smelly at times.

For a couple of days my throat became so sore and inflamed that it was difficult to speak. White blisters appeared in my mouth and down my throat. My sinuses became swollen and painful (which I had never felt before). My gums became inflamed, as if I had been through multiple dental cleanings. Each of these things happened separately, would last for a few days, and then would disappear. It seemed that my body was eliminating built up junk through my mouth, throat, and sinuses.

None of this scared me because the joint inflammation went down each day, and the joint pain diminished. My greatest wish was fulfilled—the joint pain was gone...I could handle anything else that happened. Starting with the eleventh day, my energy level was noticeably lower. I spent most of the time in my room, reading.

I was never hungry during the fast. Usually, a person is hungry for the first couple of days, until the digestive system shuts down. I was so sick when I started, that my body instinctively knew that it did not want or need food—it needed rest.

I continued the fast for fourteen days. On the fifteenth day, I was rewarded with a glass of watermelon juice. It tasted divine. The center asks that you stay and refeed for one half the number of days that you fasted. The refeeding stage is so critical. If you eat incorrectly or overeat during that initial period, you could lose some or all of the benefit that you just worked so hard for.

My taste buds were very sensitive—everything tasted incredibly good. I remember that I spat out the first bite of celery, because it tasted too salty. Celery has a high level of natural sodium, but since my taste buds had been overwhelmed with lots of table salt over the years, I didn't realize that celery tasted that way.

The first few days after the fast I was fed juice, then fruit and salad, and eventually some cooked vegetables. After a few days of eating, my energy was back and I started walking outside every day with a few other people who had completed their fasts.

I didn't just feel good, I looked good. I gained back a couple of pounds once I started eating—but was still twelve pounds lighter than when I arrived. My face had defined cheekbones, and my complexion was soft and rosy. I have a picture on my desk right now of me and two of my fasting companions. In the photo, I am smiling from ear to ear.

The fast was the most amazing thing I have ever experienced. Not only did I get rid of all the symptoms of lupus, but I now feel so empowered about all areas of my health—and the incredible self-healing power of my body.

FASTING CENTERS

These centers are experienced with medically supervised, water-only fasting.

However, several of them are also appropriate places to go to rest, recuperate, and learn how to modify your lifestyle, while eating nutritious whole vegan foods.

TrueNorth Health

Alan Goldhamer, DC
Petaluma, CA
707-586-5555
www.healthpromoting.com/Fasting/fasting.htm

This is where I fasted. Very professional, yet caring environment. Read more about TrueNorth in the fasting section, where I describe my fasting experience.

Arcadia Health Center

Alec Burton, M.Sc., D.O. Hons, D.C.
Nejla Burton, M.Sc, D.O.
Arcadia, N.S.W.
2159 Australia
www.AlecBurton.com

The two Drs. Burton have run this Center for many years and trained Dr. Goldhamer in the art of supervised fasting. I have never been to Australia, but I have met the Burtons. They are very knowledgeable and highly respected. The center is close to the city of Sydney.

Scott's Natural Health Institute

D.J. Scott, DM, ND, DC
Strongsville, Ohio
440-238-3003
www.fastingbydesign.com

Dr. Scott has run this fasting clinic for over 50 years and has fasted thousands of people. You can call Dr. Scott to discuss your situation, to determine if this center is a good fit for you.

Part Six: Recipes

MEAL SUGGESTIONS

Breakfast

Starting the day with fruit for breakfast is a big step towards getting your fresh food in! A lot of people feel better and have more energy by just eating fruit in the morning. I wake up in the morning, drink a couple of glasses of water, do some form of exercise, take a shower and then eat a fruit breakfast.

Smoothies are my favorite breakfast. I usually use two to three bananas, plus strawberries or blueberries or peaches (frozen if they're not in season). I add about 1/2 cup of water so the drink is not too thick—and if the fruit was not frozen, I add a few ice cubes. To make it even thicker, add frozen banana. (Bananas are easier to digest and taste the best when they are ripe...so you want some brown spots on the skin—not brown bruises, but brown freckles).

Believe it not, I also add fresh leafy greens; lettuce, kale, or chard. Sounds gross, but tastes good. You can start with just a few leaves, and work up to larger handfuls.

Some mornings I'll eat just sliced fresh fruit. If I'm in a hurry, I'll take fruit with me and eat it on the way.

When fruit is ripe and ready to eat—it's sweet. Some people don't like fruit because the type they buy is tasteless. Usually this is because the fruit is either not ripe, or it's been commercially versus organically grown. Commercial fruit is tasteless because it's over-watered, grown with artificial fertilizers, and picked green and artificially ripened. Whenever possible buy locally grown, and preferably organic, foods at farmer's markets.

Try papaya with a little lime squeezed on it (it's ripe when it's a bit soft when you squeeze it). Of course, apples are always good. If you're really hungry, you could eat some raw walnuts or almonds or sunflower seeds with apple. Any fresh fruit that you like is fine.

Most people who are hungry after eating just fruit in the morning, are hungry because they didn't eat enough calories. A pound of fruit has about three-hundred calories, so eat enough for your caloric needs.

When eating a lot of fruit, it's good to also eat some leafy greens or celery along with it. The greens help to balance the absorption of the fruit sugar into your bloodstream.

If you're really hungry, another good whole food breakfast is cooked oatmeal. When starting out, and you want to calm down inflammation, it's probably best to leave the oatmeal out. Oatmeal itself does not contain gluten, but most manufacturing plants that process oats also process other foods that do contain gluten. Therefore, the oatmeal you buy can contain gluten, which is a substance that a lot of people are allergic to.

Oatmeal is a food that you might be able to eat after the inflammation has cooled down. When cooking it, add cinnamon and apple pie spice. I also top the bowl off with chopped apple, and a few raisins and walnuts...it tastes like apple pie.

Lunch or dinner
- Fruit salads
- Vegetable salads
- Casseroles
- Soups
- Baked potatoes and squashes
- Brown rice dishes
- Bean dishes

Desserts

As you've probably figured out by now—ice cream isn't a whole food. It's a very processed food, full of white sugar and dairy. It's the ultimate seductive combination of sugar and fat. Remember that no food in nature is this intense with fat and sugar.

Think that you'll miss ice cream? The good news is that banana ice cream (made with frozen bananas) is really, really good and is a whole food. You could even make banana/strawberry or blueberry ice cream, and it's nutritious enough to be a meal!

In the following pages, you'll see that there are many delicious dessert recipes.

RECIPES

The following recipes are primarily made with whole food ingredients. You can omit any of the spices, onions or garlic if desired, and still have some great tasting, simple recipes.

Be sure to go to **www.LupusRecoveryDiet.com/recipes** and sign up to receive even more recipes and tips to make whole foods easy and delicious.

Beverages

"Milks"

Almond milk
2 ounces raw, finely ground almonds (1/2 cup)
1 cup water

Blend for two minutes, no need to strain.

Banana milk—great on cereal!
1 banana
½ to ¾ cup water
¼ teaspoon vanilla (optional)

Blend until smooth. Use more or less water, depending on the thickness you like.

Rice milk
1 cup cooked brown rice (still warm is best)
3 cups water
½ teaspoon vanilla
2 soaked dates (optional)

Blend for 5 minutes, until smooth. Let sit for 5 minutes. Pour into another container, being careful to not let the sediment in the bottom of the blender pour out. Can also use a strainer.

Smoothies (all ingredients are raw)

Basic Banana Smoothie
1 to 4 bananas
Handful of fresh or frozen fruit
½ cup of water (or more, depending on the thickness you like)
Few ice cubes (optional)

Add ice and fruit first to a blender, followed by bananas and then water. Blend all until smooth. The number of bananas depends on how hungry you are, and whether this is a snack or a meal.

Adding ice or frozen fruit changes the texture. Frozen banana will make this drink creamier.

Use any fruits you like—a few suggestions:
Strawberry
Blueberry
Peach
Raspberry
Papaya
Orange
Pineapple
Tangerine
Cherry
Mango
Mango & Orange
Mango & Pineapple
Peach & blueberry
Strawberry & blueberry
Orange & pineapple
Pineapple & papaya

Basic Fruit Smoothie (without banana)
2 cups fruit, fresh or frozen
½ - ¾ cup water or freshly squeezed juice
ice—if using fresh fruit

Blend. Has more of a sherbet texture than a smoothie with banana.

Fresh Juices

These are fun drinks—but optional, and not required for health. They do require a juicer.

Carrot Juice
8 to 10 carrots

Carrot-Broccoli
1 head of broccoli
5 carrots

Carrot-Celery Apple
7 carrots
3 celery stalks
1 apple

Celery Apple
8 celery stalks
1 apple

Celery Lemon
10 celery stalks
½ lemon

Apple Celery Kale
3 apples
2 celery stalks
4 kale leaves

Lemonade
4 apples
¼ lemon with skin
Serve over crushed ice

Pink Lady
¼ ripe pineapple
1 pint strawberries
1 red sweet apple
1 tart apple
Juice the apples. Blend with the pineapple until smooth. Then blend in the strawberries.

Green Drink - Cucumber Celery
1 cucumber
4 stalks celery
Very smooth and calming drink.

Salad Dressings

For a simple dressing, just squeeze the juice of an orange, lemon or lime on a salad.

Diced avocado and tomato tossed on top of a salad is also simple and delicious.

Balsamic vinegar or rice vinegar are also easy dressings.

Ground flax seed—sprinkle on top of salads and blend in smoothies. Grind whole flax seeds for 15 seconds in a small coffee bean grinder. You can grind a large batch and freeze (great source of Omega 3).

Mango Dressing—my favorite
Blend:
1 Asian mango
1 teaspoon water

Mango Orange Dressing
Blend:
1 mango (asian mango works best)
1 orange—either juiced or whole

Tomato Walnut
Blend:
2 tomatoes
2 ounces raw walnuts

Tomato Basil
1-2 tomatoes
fresh basil
fresh lemon juice

Blend tomatoes with lemon juice. Stir in chopped basil. Add a little water if needed. Can add ¼ avocado for creamier texture.

Lemon Tahini
Blend:
4 ounces raw tahini (sesame butter)
3 ounces of water
1 peeled lemon.
 2 dates, softened by soaking in water (optional)

Avocado Tomato
Blend:
2 tomatoes
1 avocado
1 tablespoon fresh herb—such as dill or cilantro.

Avocado Orange
Blend:
½ avocado
1 orange or ½ cup fresh squeezed orange juice
2 tablespoons lemon juice

Fruit sauces—good on green salads or fruit salads

Strawberry-Banana Sauce
Blend:
12 strawberries
1 banana
squeeze of orange juice

Pear Sauce—good on bananas
Blend:
Pears
Water
2 dates (optional)

Salads

Make salad preparation easy—create a refrigerator salad bar:

Wash leafy lettuce (don't use iceberg, it has no nutrients) and chard in a good quality salad spinner (the XO brand is a good one). A good salad spinner is airtight and you can store the lettuce in it—keeping it fresh and crispy.

Set up containers with shredded carrots, sliced cucumber, diced celery, diced peppers and diced tomatoes. It's very quick and easy to create a colorful salad this way.

Vegetable Salads

Cole Slaw
4 cups cabbage, shredded
2 cups carrots, shredded
Toss with a nut dressing, fruit sauce, or vinegar.

Blended salads
Just put your salad in a food processor or blender. A food processor gives more of a leafy texture, while the blender produces more of a soup-like texture. Use any combination of lettuce, broccoli, celery, red pepper, kale, or chard. This creates a finely chopped, easy to eat salad.

You can either pour a dressing on afterwards, or add fruit while processing. Mango, apple and orange are good fruits to blend with the greens. You can also add 1/4 avocado while blending a salad.

Broccoli Cauliflower Salad
2 cups cauliflower
2 cups broccoli
2 cups cut leaf lettuce
2 cups romaine lettuce
1 tomato, chopped
1 celery stalk, chopped
¼ cup shredded zucchini

Use broccoli and cauliflower fresh or slightly steamed. Cut into small pieces. Combine everything in a bowl and toss with nut butter or other dressing.

Pea Salad

2 cups sugar snap peas
1 cup raw corn
1 cup chopped cucumber
1 cup grated cabbage
½ cup chopped red pepper

Toss together and garnish with sprouts (broccoli sprouts, not alfalfa).

Stuffed Tomatoes

Lettuce Leaves
1 tomato
½ - 1 cup of rice salad

Slice the tomato in six sections, nearly to the base. Arrange lettuce on a plate. Place tomato in center of the plate and fill the center with the salad.

Pepper Bowls

Cut red or yellow pepper in half, removing seeds. Line with lettuce or sprouts, and stuff with a dip or blended salad.

Chopped Salad
2 carrots
2 celery stalks
1 bunch parsley
1 red or yellow pepper
4 kale leaves
1 small red onion
garbanzo beans
splash of rice vinegar

Chop all vegetables into small pieces. Mix together in bowl. Will keep for a few days.

Carrot Salad
5 carrots, shredded
3 tablespoons fresh orange juice
10 raisins, cut in half
cinnamon to taste
Mix together.
Fruit Salads

Fruit Salads

Pineapple Orange Salad
1 pineapple, skin removed and cut into small pieces
1 orange, divided into sections
1 cup strawberries, cut in half
mint leaves
Toss together.

Orange Berry Medley
Oranges and berries (strawberries, blueberries, raspberries)
1-2 ounces raw almonds or sunflower seeds
Lettuce leaves

Toss together and arrange on lettuce leaves

Melon Salad
1 honeydew
1 cantaloupe
1 watermelon

Peel and seed all melons. Cut into cubes or use a melon scoop to form small balls.

Waldorf Salad
1 red apple, chopped
1 stalk of celery, chopped
seedless grapes
romaine lettuce leaves
walnuts (optional)
Toss together.

Spreads and Dips

Use zucchini slices, carrot slices and celery sticks in place of chips for dipping into salsa, hummus, and spreads. I've even taken zucchini slices (chips) to Mexican restaurants with me, to dip in the salsa and guacamole—instead of eating oily fried chips. Other people at the table usually ask if they can have some, too.

Salsa
1 tomato, diced
1 small onion, diced
1 clove of garlic, chopped
3 tablespoons fresh cilantro, diced
2 tablespoons fresh lemon juice

Mix all ingredients together in a bowl.

Guacamole
1 avocado
1 small tomato, chopped
½ small onion, chopped
1 clove of garlic, minced
1 tablespoon lemon juice
fresh chopped cilantro (optional)

Mash avocado with a fork in a small bowl. Mix in the remaining ingredients.

Avocado Dip
Blend or mash with fork.
¼ cup juice—carrot, celery and/or red pepper
1 avocado

Bean Free Hummus
Blend:
Zucchini, peeled and cut in chunks
2 tablespoons tahini butter
2 tablespoons fresh lemon juice

Hummus (Chickpea Pate)
2 cups cooked garbanzo beans
¼ cup raw tahini
1/3 cup lemon juice
2 garlic cloves (optional)
cumin (optional)
fresh parsley or mint
¼ cup water or vegetable broth

Blend all ingredients until smooth and creamy. Add more water or lemon if needed.

Tahini-Free Hummus
2 cups cooked garbanzo beans (canned or fresh)
2 tablespoon lemon juice
1 clove garlic, minced
½ cup vegetable broth or water
pinch of cayenne pepper
1 tablespoon red onion, minced
2 tablespoons parsley, minced

Blend garbanzos, lemon, garlic, cayenne and broth until smooth and creamy. Stir in parsley and red onion. Add more water if needed.

Eggplant Pate
2 medium eggplants
1 lemon
3 tablespoons cilantro, chopped
2 tablespoons sesame seeds (optional)

Pierce eggplant multiple times with a fork. Place on pan and bake at 400 degrees for 45 to 60 minutes. The eggplant will be very soft on the inside and almost burnt looking on the outside.

Once cool enough to handle, peel off the outer skin. Mash or blend the pulp with the lemon. Stir in other ingredients. Delicious warm or room temperature.

Black Bean Dip
2 cups cooked black beans
3 tablespoons fresh lime or lemon juice
½ teaspoon garlic powder
½ teaspoon cumin powder
Pinch of cayenne or chili powder (optional)

Blend together until smooth, adding water if needed. Can also stir in a few tablespoons of fresh salsa.

Sandwiches and Wraps

Bread substitutes:
Roll up in large flat green collard leaf
Roll up in large lettuce leaf
Roll up in rice paper wrapper
Oven face sandwich on Portobello mushroom

Some sandwich suggestions: (with or without bread)
Hummus, lettuce and tomato
Avocado, lettuce and tomato
Lettuce, tomato, kale, mustard
Portobello mushroom, hummus, and eggplant
Eggplant pate

If you are eating breads and grains, some good choices are:
100% Whole grain bread
Non-gluten breads (such as brown rice bread)
Whole-wheat pita bread
Wheat or corn tortilla wraps
Corn taco shells

Soups and Stews

I love soups. You can make a pot that will last during the week, or freeze servings for later. If you don't have the energy to cook— ask a friend to make a pot for you.

You can also top potatoes, rice, vegetables or salad with soup.

Gazpacho (served cold)
6 tomatoes
1 cucumber, peeled and chopped
½ cup diced celery
1 sweet red pepper, diced
½ cup minced parsley
3 T fresh lemon juice
3 cups minced chives (optional)

Blend 3 tomatoes, ½ cucumber, ½ red pepper, ¼ cup parsley, and lemon juice. In separate bowl, combine 3 chopped tomatoes, ½ cucumber, ½ red pepper, ¼ cup parsley and chives. Stir in the blended mixture. Chill.

Lava soup (served room temperature)
12 ounces fresh carrot juice
1/2 avocado
1 tablespoon lime juice
½ t grated ginger

Blend all ingredients until smooth. Squeeze additional lime juice on top just before serving. Delicious. Can also use as a dressing by adding less juice (makes it thicker).

Vegetable Soup Stock
6 cups water
4 ribs celery, coarsely chopped
3 large carrots
1/2 bunch Swiss chard
½ bunch spinach
1 small zucchini
1 cup of mushrooms and stems (leftover stems are fine)
1 onion
1/2 bunch parsley
1 teaspoon dried thyme
1 bay leaf
6 whole cloves

Bring water to a boil. Add all ingredients. Simmer for one hour. Let the broth cool completely. Strain the broth into another large pot, pressing firmly on all the vegetables to extract as much juice as possible.

Store the broth in jars or freezer bags. You can use any vegetables, but don't use broccoli, cauliflower, brussel sprouts or any vegetable in the cabbage family (their flavor is too strong). Don't use potatoes as they absorb the flavors of the other vegetables.

Easy Vegetable Soup
Leftover steamed veggies
Vegetable juice, vegetable broth or vegetables blended with water for the stock.

Heat and serve.

Green Velvet Soup, from Jennifer Raymond's *Fat Free and Easy Cookbook*
This beautiful soup is a delicious way to eat green vegetables.

1 onion, chopped
2 celery stalks, sliced
2 potatoes, scrubbed and diced
¾ cup split peas, rinsed
2 bay leaves
6 cups water or vegetable stock
2 medium zucchini, diced
1 medium stalk broccoli, chopped
1 bunch fresh spinach, washed and chopped
½ teaspoon basil
¼ teaspoon black pepper

Place the onion, celery, potatoes, split peas, and bay leaves in a large pot with water or stock and bring to a boil. Reduce heat to low, cover, and simmer 1 hour. Remove the bay leaves.

Add the zucchini, broccoli, spinach, basil, and black pepper. Simmer 20 minutes. Transfer to a blender in several small batches and blend until completely smooth, holding the lid on tightly. (You can also use a hand blender and blend the soup in the pot.) Return to the pot and heat until steamy. Serves 10.

Butternut Squash Soup
1 butternut squash (about 1 ¾ pounds)
4-½ cups water or vegetable broth
1 teaspoon curry powder
½ teaspoon black pepper
2 handfuls of washed spinach

Peel the butternut squash, and cut into chunks. Cut out the seeds and pulp. Place the squash in a large pot along with the broth. Bring to a boil, then lower heat and add the curry powder and pepper. Simmer for 30 minutes, or until the squash is tender when poked with a fork.

Blend the squash and liquid together and return it to the pot. Stir in the spinach and simmer for another 5 minutes before serving.

Sweet Potato Soup
2 ½ cups water or vegetable stock
1 onion chopped
2 garlic cloves, minced
4 large sweet potatoes or yams, peeled and cut into chunks
½ head broccoli
½ head cauliflower
4 chard leaves
6 mushrooms (optional)

Place sweet potato and vegetables in a soup pot. Fill the pot with soup stock, just covering the chopped vegetables. Bring to a boil and simmer until all ingredients are well cooked (about 30 minutes). Blend.

Lentil Soup
1 cup dried lentils
5 cups water or vegetable broth
2 cloves garlic, minced
½ cup onion, chopped
1 carrot, chopped

1 tablespoon basil
1 tablespoon parsley flakes
2 tomatoes, chopped (or 1 can)
4-6 cups spinach or kale, chopped (or use frozen)

Bring water to a boil in large saucepan. Add lentils, basil, parsley, carrot, onion and garlic. Simmer for 30 minutes. Then add the greens and tomatoes and simmer for 30 more minutes. For a thicker soup, blend 1/3 and return it to the pot
(For a curried lentil soup, can add 1 teaspoon whole cumin seeds with the lentils and 1 teaspoon curry powder when adding the spinach.)

Garbanzo and Cabbage Soup
6 teaspoons water
1 onion, chopped
1 garlic clove, chopped
1 cup chopped tomato, fresh or canned
4 cups chopped cabbage
1 potato, diced
¼ cup chopped parsley
4 cups water or vegetable stock
2 cups cooked garbanzo beans, fresh or canned
1 teaspoon black pepper
1 teaspoon paprika

Heat the water, garlic, paprika and pepper in a large pot and sauté the onion a few minutes until soft. Add the tomato, cabbage, potato, water or stock, and garbanzo beans. Simmer until the cabbage and potato are tender, about 20 minutes.

Blend 3 cups of the soup and return it to the pot (or partially blend in the pot with a hand blender).

Sauces—for vegetables, potatoes, rice, or squash.

Leftover Veggie Sauce
Blend any leftover veggies together with a small amount of water or vegetable broth. Pour over vegetables, potatoes or rice.

Creamy Sauce

Blend small amount of nut butter with a main ingredient—tomato, cucumber, fresh vegetables, steamed vegetables. Add water or carrot or beet juice to get the right consistency.

Vegetable Sauce

1 whole steamed zucchini
1 whole yam or sweet potato
1 whole white potato

Place all in blender (zucchini first). Blend until smooth.

Quick Garbanzo Gravy

1 cup chopped onion
¼ teaspoon low-sodium tamari (it's like soy sauce)
1-½ cups cooked garbanzo beans (or 1 can)
¼ teaspoon poultry seasoning

Braise onions by heating onions, soy sauce and ¼ cup of water in saucepan until liquid evaporates. Add another ¼ cup of water and let that also evaporate. Add ¼ cup water, and stir to loosen onion pieces from the bottom of the pan. Put in blender. Add garbanzos, the seasoning, and 1 cup of water or vegetable broth. Blend.

Tomato Sauce

3 cups chopped tomato
¼ cup chopped parsley
4 tablespoons lemon juice
½ teaspoon basil
½ teaspoon rosemary
1 garlic clove, minced or 1 teaspoon garlic powder
2 tablespoons chopped onion

Put onions, garlic and a few tablespoons of water in a large skillet, and stir sauté until soft. Stir in the chopped tomatoes and remaining ingredients. Simmer over low heat for 15 minutes, stirring occasionally.

The Basics

Brown Rice
To cook rice, I recommend using a kitchen appliance called a steamer. It is virtually foolproof. I plug it in, mix one cup of rice and 1 and ½ cups of water, turn the timer to 60 minutes—go play tennis and the rice is perfectly done when I return. You can buy a steamer for about $30—be sure it has the capacity to steam rice, as well as vegetables. Black and Decker has several models.

If you don't have a steamer—here's an easy way to cook rice, so that it doesn't get too dry:

1 cup short or long grain brown rice
4 cups water

Rinse and drain the rice. Bring the water to a boil in a saucepan, and then add the rice. Once the water returns to a boil, lower the heat slightly, then cover loosely and boil gently about 40 minutes, until the rice is soft but still retains a hint of crunchiness. Pour off any excess liquid. (This liquid can be saved and used as a broth for soups and stews if desired.)

Baked Potato
Wash the skin of a russet potato under running water. Pierce with a knife to release steam. Place in 375-degree oven. Bake for 1 hour or until tender to the touch.

Baked Sweet Potato
Wash the skin of a yam or sweet potato under running water. (I prefer the Japanese sweet potato—it's white inside). Do not pierce with a knife—the potato will leak while cooking. Cook at 375 degrees for about fifty minutes, or until tender to the touch.

Baked Squash
Butternut squash
Acorn squash

Bake in 350 degree oven for 1-½ hours or until a fork can be easily inserted. Cool and then cut in half, removing seeds. Serve as is, or scoop out the flesh from the skin and stuff with brown rice or vegetables.

You can also cook squash by cutting it half lengthwise and placing it cut side down on a baking pan. It probably cooks faster and more evenly when cut before cooking. However, some people have difficulty cutting through an uncooked squash—and in that case, cooking it whole is best.

Steamed Vegetables
Vegetables can either be "steamed" or "stir-fried." To steam vegetables, add about 1 inch of water to a large saucepan. Insert a metal "steamer basket". Place the vegetables in the basket, so that they are not touching the water. Steam covered, at a slow boil—not too hot.

Steam the vegetables for as short a time as possible—usually 3-5 minutes is plenty—depending on the vegetable. The goal is for the vegetables to be slightly tender, without becoming overcooked and mushy.

Quinoa (fast cooking and delicious grain)
Place 1 cup quinoa and 2 cups water in a saucepan and bring to a boil. Reduce the heat to simmer, cover and cook until all the water is absorbed (10-15 minutes). When done, the quinoa will be soft and translucent looking.

Oatmeal
Bring 1 ½ cups of water to a boil in a small saucepan (I add ½ teaspoon cinnamon or apple pie spice to the water). Add ¾ cups of rolled oats and simmer for about 12 minutes, until water is absorbed. Cover; turn off heat and let sit for 3 minutes.

Oatmeal is not thought to contain gluten—but often has traces of gluten from the processing plant, which is also processing glutinous grains. If you are on a gluten-free diet, it's best to not eat oatmeal.

Beans

Beans are easy to cook, but require a little advanced planning. Rinse the beans and soak for 6 to 8 hours. Drain the beans, add fresh water and cook on the stovetop until tender.

Soaking is not required, but it makes the beans easier to digest. You can freeze beans to use later.

The following chart is from Jennifer Raymond's *The Peaceful Palate* cookbook.

Beans	Water	Cook Time	Yield
black beans	3 cups	1-½ hours	2¼ cup
garbanzos	4 cups	2 hours	2½ cups
lentils, brown	3 cups	1 hour	2 ¼ cups
lentils, orange	3 cups	20 minutes	2cups
navy beans	3 cups	1 ½ hour	2 cups
split peas	3 cups	1 hour	2½ cups

Vegetables

Buy your vegetables for the week, cut them up into bite-sized pieces and store them in Ziploc bags in the refrigerator. You can just pull out a bunch of bags and create a steamed veggie plate in a few minutes. Steam vegetables until just tender, so that they retain more of their nutrients.

Steamed Broccoli and or Cauliflower
Good mixed with rice with a sauce on top (see sauces).

Spinach
Steamed with a little garlic. Topped with lemon.

Brussel Sprouts
Slice in half and steam for about 12 minutes or until tender. Serve with dip, spread or sauce.

Green beans with braised onions
Heat up a few tablespoons of water. Add onions and minced garlic. Cook until water is evaporated. Add a few more tablespoons of water and cook again until water is evaporated. The longer you do this, the more caramelized the onions become.

Steam green beans for 15-20 minutes or until tender and stir in warm braised onions.

Braised / Steamed Kale or Swiss Kale
Freshly steamed or braised Swiss chard has a delicious naturally salty flavor. Mix some steamed chard with some mashed baked potatoes.

Baked Broccoli, Cauliflower, Bell Pepper, Onion and Sweet Potato
Break broccoli and cauliflower into florets. Chop pepper, onion and potato into small chunks. Toss in a bowl with a little water, rosemary and garlic powder. Place on baking sheet and roast in the oven at 375-degrees for 25-30 minutes. Tastes very different than when steamed.

Cabbage
1 onion
4 cups shredded (chopped) cabbage
1 teaspoon cumin

Heat 6 tablespoons of water and sauté the onion and cumin until soft (about 4 minutes). Add the shredded cabbage and stir. Simmer cabbage for about 15 minutes until tender. In place of cumin, use any spices you like—such as Indian, Mexican, or Thai.

Potatoes

Twice Baked Potatoes
Bake a potato. Cut in half, lengthwise. Scoop out the pulp, leaving a thin layer of potato on the outer skin. Mash the pulp with a little water, cooked sweet potato, and garlic. Stuff the potato back into the skins, and heat at 400-degrees for a few

more minutes, until the skins are slightly crunchy. Garnish with diced green onion.

French Fries
Slice russet potatoes into rounds. Cut the rounds into 4 or 6 pieces. Toss these pieces with garlic and/or onion powder. Place on a baking sheet lined with parchment paper and bake at 400-degrees for 15 minutes. Turn the potatoes over and bake for another 10 minutes. Serve with salsa or ketchup. Yummy!

Mashed Potatoes
Peel potatoes and cut into chunks. Steam or boil for 15-20 minutes, until tender. Mash with water, vegetable broth or rice milk. Roasted garlic added to this is delicious (see spreads).

Main Dishes

Really, most of the recipes in this book can be considered a main dish, when served with a salad. That's what great about whole foods...

Brown Rice and Vegetables—traditional, simple favorite. Top with a sauce.

Spaghetti Squash
1 spaghetti squash
 tomato sauce (home made or an oil-free bottled sauce)

Bake squash at 350 degrees for 1 hour or until tender to the touch. Cool slightly. Cut in half lengthwise—and using a fork, scrape the inner flesh of the squash. It will be stringy and look like long strands of pasta.

Put on plate and pour tomato sauce on top. Delicious, it really looks and tastes like pasta.

Stuffed Acorn Squash
Cut in half lengthwise. Place cut side down in a baking dish, along with a little water. Cook at 375-degrees for one hour, or

until tender. Scoop out the seeds and pulp. Stuff the opening with wild rice mixed with spinach.

Quinoa Casserole

1 cup quinoa
2 cups water or vegetable broth
½ cup diced carrots
½ cup diced celery
½ cup diced red pepper
½ cup diced green beans
½ cup diced green pepper

Rinse and wash quinoa two times. Combine all ingredients in large saucepan and cook for 10-15 minutes, or until all the water is absorbed. Can top with vegetable sauce when serving.

Grilled Eggplant Patties

Slice eggplant in rounds. Sauté for 1 minute in balsamic vinegar and minced garlic. Grill on stovetop in nonstick pan or on outdoor grill.

Grilled Portobello Mushrooms

Marinate in balsamic vinegar and minced garlic for 30 seconds. Cook on outdoor grill or stovetop skillet. Can also grill red peppers at the same time. Delicious together. Spread layer of hummus on top of mushroom, and top with roasted red pepper (I won an outdoor grill contest with this one).

Grilled Vegetable Kabob

Mushroom
Green or red pepper
Chunks of onion
Garlic powder

Marinate vegetables in balsamic vinegar for 1 minute. Sprinkle with garlic powder. Skewer and place on outdoors grill. If eating soy, can add chunks of firm tofu on the skewer.

Desserts   Many of these desserts contain all "raw" ingredients—no cooking involved.

Banana "ice cream"

Peel ripe bananas. Slice in half lengthwise. Freeze in plastic bags for at least four hours. Before using, let the bananas defrost for 10-15 minutes. Cut into smaller chunks and place in a food processor with the S blade. Process until the texture is the consistency of ice cream.

You can also add frozen fruit—blueberry or peach ice cream are my two favorites (Use a Champion Juicer to get a great consistency). Pour a fruit sauce over top, or sprinkle with fresh fruit and nuts. You won't believe how much it tastes like ice cream!!

Banana Popsicles

Peel ripe banana and insert a wooden Popsicle stick in the end. Leave plain or roll in nuts or coconut or carob powder. Freeze.

Frozen Juice Pops

Pour freshly squeezed juice in Popsicle holders. Get creative and add fresh fruit too!

Fresh Dates

Fresh dates are a delicious sweet treat by themselves. You can also split a date in half and add raw almonds or raw nut butter.

Sherbet

8 frozen strawberries
1 large peeled frozen banana
1 medium mango, peeled and cubed, frozen

Blend each individually with a little fresh squeezed orange juice. Serve over a bed of lettuce and fruit salad

Part Seven: Resources

"When setting out on a journey, never consult someone who has never left home"

—Rumi, 1207-1273 A.D

HIGHLY RECOMMENDED BOOKS

These books are essential reading, and are all available in public libraries.

The China Study
T. Colin Campbell, PhD

Prevent and Reverse Heart Disease
Caldwell B. Esselyton, M.D.

McDougall's Medicine, A Challenging Second Opinion
John A. McDougall, M.D.

Fasting and Eating for Health
Joel Fuhrman, M.D.

RETREAT CENTERS

In addition to the fasting centers listed in the fasting section, these are retreat centers that people refer to in their personal stories.

Arcadia Health Center

Alec Burton, M.Sc., D.O. Hons, D.C.
Nejla Burton, M.Sc, D.O.
Arcadia, N.S.W.
2159 Australia
www.AlecBurton.com

McDougall Live In Program

John McDougall, M.D.
Santa Rosa, CA
www.drmcdougall.com
drmcdougall@drmcdougall.com
800-941-7111

Scott's Natural Health Institute

D.J. Scott, DM, ND, DC
Strongsville, Ohio
440-238-3003
www.fastingbydesign.com

TrueNorth Health

Alan Goldhamer, DC
Petaluma, CA
707-586-5555
www.healthpromoting.com

Uchee Pines
Agatha Thrash, MD
Seale, Alabama
334-855-4764
www.UcheePines.org

Weimar Institute / NEWSTART® **Program**
Weimar, California
800-525-9192
www.Weimar.org

REFERENCES

Bernard, Neal MD, Foods That Fight Pain

Cridland, Ronald MD, Natural Hygiene Care vs. Medical Management, *Health Science*, May/June 1997

Cridland, Ronald MD, Your Health Depends on Sleep, *Health Science*, Nov/Dec 1993

Cridland, Ronald MD, Dietary Excess: Prescription for Poor Health, *Health Science* Jan/Feb 1993

Editors of Health Science Magazine, *A Natural Hygiene Handbook*, American Natural Hygiene Society, 1996

Eisman, George, M.A. Msc., R.D., *A Basic Course in Vegetarian and Vegan Nutrition*, New York, Diet-Ethics Books, Eighth Edition Revised, 2003

Fuhrman M.D., Joel *Eat to Live*, Boston, Little Brown and Company, 2003

Goldhamer D.C., Alan, *The Health Promoting Cookbook*, Summertown, Book Publishing Company, 1997

Goldhamer, Alan *Where do you get your protein? Everything you need to know about this frequently asked question* (www.healthpromoting.com/Articles/articles.htm).

Havala, Suzanne, The Complete Idiot's Guide to Being Vegetarian, Alpha Books, 1999

Lahita M.D., Robert G. and Phillips, PhD, Robert H., *Lupus: Everything You Need to Know*, New York, Avery Publishing, 1998

Lisle PhD, Douglas J and Goldhamer D.C., Alan *The Pleasure Trap*, Healthy Living Publications, 2003

McDougall M.D., John A, *McDougall's Medicine, A Challenging Second Opinion*, New Win Publishing, 1985

McDougall M.D., John A., The McDougall Program, Twelve Days to Dynamic Health, NAL Books, 1990

McDougall J, article, *Diet, The Only Hope for Arthritis* (www.drmcdougall.com).

Raymond, Jennifer, *The Peaceful Palate,* Heart and Soul Publications, 1996

Raymond, Jennifer, *Fat-Free and Easy*, Heart and Soul Publications, 1997

Saunders, Kerrie K., *The Vegan Diet as Chronic Disease Prevention*, New York, Lantern Books, 2003

Spock M.D., Benjamin and Parker M.D., Steven, *Dr. Spock's Baby and Child Care*, 7th edition, New York, Penguin Group, 1998

Wallace, Daniel J, *The Lupus Book*, New York, Oxford University Press, 2000

Wallace, Daniel J, and Wallace, Janice B, *Making Sense of Fibromyalgia*, Oxford University Press, 1999

There's Lots More at Jill's Website...

Go to Jill's website at www.LupusRecoveryDiet.com/recipes to get more FREE recipes that make eating whole foods easy and delicious!

You'll also scc additional resources on the website; articles, audio books, cookbooks, videos, kitchen supplies, and more...

www.LupusRecoveryDiet.com/recipes

Made in the USA
Columbia, SC
31 May 2019